Move for Moo

Move for Mood

The Psychology of Exercise
How movement directly influences emotions and cognitive performance.

Dr. Adrian Vale

Mindful Pages

Published in 2025

ISBN: 9789371773065 (PB)
ISBN: 9789371777490 (eBook)

Published by

Mindful Pages
Imprint of Alpha Editions LLC
312 W. 2nd St #1834
Casper, WY 82601, USA

This book was developed using advanced writing tools to support the drafting and ideation process. All content has been thoughtfully curated, refined, and reviewed to ensure quality and relevance.

Content

Introduction
Movement as Mind

Within psychology, movement has too often been treated as an afterthought—a supporting mechanism, useful perhaps, but secondary to the so-called higher functions of mind and language. This hierarchy, so deeply ingrained in Western thought, has always been a little suspect, and today it is growing impossible to defend. What happens if we invert it? If we treat movement not as background noise but as a primary medium of knowing and feeling, a language in which mind and body converse seamlessly? *Move for Mood: The Psychology of Exercise* takes precisely this stance. Here, movement is not framed as a supplement to mental health but as a form of intelligence in its own right, an embodied grammar through which thought, mood, and identity emerge.

For centuries, the cognitive model has dominated psychology, placing its trust in processes like reasoning, memory, and linguistic reflection. Valuable though they are, these processes tell only half the story. The body is not a neutral courier of consciousness, ferrying the mind from room to room. It shapes, colours, and even originates much of what we call thought. Movement is a voice, subtle yet insistent, articulating emotion, identity, and presence with every gesture and rhythm. To ignore this dimension is to flatten human experience, to dismiss the layered dialogue of nerves, muscles, and brain from which our emotional lives are spun.

This book seeks to overturn that lingering Cartesian divide which carves mind away from body. It suggests, instead, that the body is a living text—a repository of memory and affect, a speaker in its own right. Posture, rhythm, and gesture are not symbolic afterthoughts but living inscriptions of psychological truth. When we learn to listen to that voice, we discover forms of knowledge inaccessible to the purely verbal mind. The body is not merely echoing emotion; it is generating it.

Such arguments gain particular urgency in our present cultural moment. Modern life, with its endless screens, desk-bound routines, and fractured attention, has left many in a state of estrangement from their physical selves. The consequences are visible everywhere: rising anxiety, low-grade depression, chronic stress, a general sense of dislocation. Against this backdrop, reclaiming movement is not simply a recommendation for better health; it is a necessity for psychological survival. To move again, attentively and with presence, is to re-open a channel of emotional coherence that contemporary life has all but closed.

It must be said, though, that *Move for Mood* is not another exercise manual, nor is it dressed up in the tired rhetoric of motivational slogans. It is a sustained investigation into the psychology of movement itself—an invitation to re-enter the body as a space of meaning, a site of emotional intelligence. The exploration here is layered, pulling from neuroscience, somatic psychology, cultural studies, and lived testimony. Readers encounter research alongside narrative case studies, interspersed with reflective practices designed to sharpen awareness of how movement sculpts mood and identity.

One of the central shifts the book encourages is a reframing of exercise. Instead of chasing instrumental goals—weight loss, endurance, efficiency—movement is recast as a practice of presence, of listening as much as doing. It becomes a kind of literacy, an embodied fluency that allows us to read ourselves more fully. Cultural norms, technological dependencies, even the personal stories we tell about discipline and self-worth—each of these has shaped our relationship with motion. To interrogate and re-imagine that relationship is, in many respects, to renegotiate the terms of our inner lives.

Emerging research strengthens this perspective. The field of embodied cognition demonstrates that thought is not confined to grey matter but springs from sensory-motor processes.

Neuroscience reveals how rhythmic movement synchronises networks in the brain that govern mood and adaptability. Somatic therapies show us how trauma inscribes itself as frozen movement, and how recovery often requires restoring physical rhythm. These findings converge on a single truth: mental health is inseparable from embodied life.

Still, theory alone would be dry. The book insists on practice. It guides readers to attend to the subtler registers of their bodies—the weight carried in a shoulder, the breath that quickens before a thought, the small shift in gait that says more than words. Movement here is not abstracted from culture but embedded in it: in ritual, in metaphor, in communal expression. To reclaim one's bodily intelligence is, in part, to resist the commodification of the body that modern culture so aggressively enforces.

Thus *Move for Mood* gestures towards a psychology that begins not with cerebral abstractions but with motion itself. It invites us to reconsider what emotion and selfhood mean when we pay heed to the body's silent eloquence. Grounded in science yet attentive to the poetry of lived experience, it seeks not only to broaden our understanding but to alter our manner of living in body and mind alike.

What you will not find here are quick fixes, nor the promise of tidy regimens. Instead, the book sketches a map—an intricate one—for navigating the inner terrain by way of the body's natural rhythms. It calls the reader into a fuller way of being, where psychology ceases to be the chatter of the mind alone and is lived instead in the pulse of breath, the cadence of steps, the arc of a stretch. And perhaps, just perhaps, your next true insight will not come through thought at all, but through the movement you didn't know was already teaching you.

Chapter 1
The Motion Mind

The prevailing picture of cognition has long been that of the brain, sealed within its bony vault, spinning the threads of thought, language, and abstract reasoning while the body obediently trails behind as servant and executor. Such a division—so comfortably entrenched in Western philosophy and the history of psychology—has concealed a far more intricate reality. Cognition is not confined to the cerebral cortex alone but is born of an ongoing, dynamic exchange between brain, body, and environment. This chapter begins from that premise, tracing how muscles, limbs, and physical rhythms are not peripheral but central scaffolding in the architecture of thought and feeling, rooting the life of the mind firmly in the textures of movement.

The theory of embodied cognition unsettles the long-held notion that thinking happens exclusively in the neural circuitry of the skull. Instead, it insists that perception and action—the sensory-motor exchanges through which we navigate the world—are not auxiliary but constitutive of memory, concept formation, and emotional regulation. Abstract reasoning, far from being detached or ethereal, is shaped by the lived encounter of the body with its surroundings. Consider posture and gait: research shows that a drooping stance is strongly linked with states of sadness or exhaustion, while an upright bearing tends to accompany alertness and confidence. Such bodily expressions are not after-the-fact signatures of mood; they participate actively in moulding how emotions surface and develop.

At the neural level, the case grows even more compelling. Oscillations in the brain—those rhythmic surges of electrical activity—do not beat on in isolation. They fall into step with the cadences of the body. Walking, dancing, even repetitive hand gestures can entrain neural networks governing mood, attention, and creative problem-solving. Movement, then, is not merely output from the brain but a subtle instrument for tuning its inner harmonies. A steady walking rhythm or the synchrony of a dance sequence aligns oscillations in ways that expand flexibility of thought and stabilise emotional states. It is little wonder that rhythmic movement and body-based therapies have found success in alleviating depression, anxiety, and cognitive decline.

Yet how peculiar, and perhaps troubling, that stillness has come to be so revered in modern cultures—as a symbol of focus, self-control, or discipline. For the vast majority of human history, motion was our natural condition. To hunt, to forage, to migrate—survival demanded a life in motion. These continual engagements with the environment did not merely sustain bodies but also exercised minds. With industrialisation and, more recently, digital immersion, the rhythm has been broken. Static postures, desk-bound work, and endless screens have alienated the brain from the bodily feedback it evolved to expect. Unsurprisingly, many researchers now speak of a crisis, an epidemic of disembodiment underlying the rising tide of mental health difficulties in our time.

But it is not only the grand gestures—the striding, the running—that matter. The tiny, half-forgotten movements of everyday life tell their own story. A restless tap of the foot, a slight hunch of the shoulders, the unconscious play of the hands: these are not idle quirks but embodied signals, often surfacing before awareness catches up. The tapping may betray an undercurrent of anxiety; a clenched jaw, the anger one cannot voice. Neuroscience suggests that such micro-movements are more than symptoms: they feed back into the emotional system, shaping experience in real time. To learn their language is to unlock new layers of self-knowledge and emotional regulation, recognising the body not as mute vessel but as active partner in the psyche's work.

By rooting cognition in motion, this chapter sets the foundation for a reconfigured vision of mind—one in which body and thought are not separate domains but reciprocal forces, endlessly shaping one another. It asks the reader to put aside inherited assumptions about the origins of mental life and to glimpse instead the intricate dialogue of nerve, muscle, and feeling that composes the fabric of experience. What follows is an invitation: to see how embodied cognition reshapes familiar psychological theories, how rhythmic motion orchestrates the brain's inner music, and how the smallest gestures can reveal entire landscapes of the self. This interweaving of neuroscience, psychology, and somatic insight points towards a striking realisation: movement is not incidental to mental health—it is its ground and genesis.

Embodied Brain

The notion that cognition is primarily a function of the brain, confined within the cranial vault and detached from the body's movements, has long shaped Western scientific and philosophical thought. Yet, this perspective overlooks a fundamental truth that has gained increasing validation: *cognition begins not in isolation but in the muscles, through the sensory-motor interactions that weave the body and mind into an inseparable whole.* The theory of embodied cognition challenges entrenched dualisms, asserting that sensory and motor systems do more than support thinking—they constitute the very substrate of thought and emotion. Far from being mere executors of mental commands, our muscles, postures, and gestures play a formative role in shaping how we perceive, reason, and regulate our emotions.

One need only observe the subtle interplay between movement and mood to recognise this intimate connection. Clinical psychologists have long noted how posture influences emotional state: an upright, open posture often correlates with feelings of confidence and optimism, while slumped shoulders tend to accompany sadness or low energy. Such observations, once dismissed as anecdotal, are now backed by rigorous empirical studies. For example, research published in *Psychological Science* demonstrates that adopting expansive postures can increase feelings of power and reduce cortisol levels—biological markers of stress—thereby actively shaping affective experience. This lends credence to the proposition that the body is not simply a container for the mind but a dynamic participant in the construction of psychological states.

The implications of embodied cognition extend beyond posture to encompass gait—the rhythmic pattern of walking. Studies employing motion capture and neuroimaging reveal that gait does not simply reflect internal mood but modulates it. In one notable experiment, participants asked to walk with longer strides and an elevated chin reported increased feelings of happiness and alertness compared to those adopting shuffling, downward-looking walks.

Gait, it seems, functions as a feedback loop: the way we move influences how we feel, which in turn shapes subsequent movement, creating a continuous dialogue between body and mind. This cyclical relationship disrupts the conventional top-down model of cognition, where the brain directs the body as a separate tool.

Underlying this interplay is the brain's remarkable plasticity and integration of sensory-motor information. Neuroscientific advances have revealed extensive bidirectional pathways connecting motor regions with those responsible for emotion and cognition. The premotor cortex, traditionally associated with planning movement, also activates during tasks requiring social understanding and empathy, suggesting a shared neural basis for action and affective cognition. Mirror neurons, discovered in the 1990s, further illuminate how observing others' movements evokes corresponding activity in the observer's motor system, underpinning processes such as imitation, learning, and emotional resonance. This neurological architecture underscores the primacy of movement not just as physical activity but as a core language of cognition.

The embodied brain's reliance on movement also extends to the domain of memory and conceptual thought. Contrary to earlier views that considered abstract thinking detached from bodily experience, current evidence reveals that sensorimotor systems are recruited even during ostensibly 'pure' cognitive tasks. Functional MRI studies demonstrate activation of motor areas when subjects imagine manipulating objects or engage with action-related language. This means that the very concepts we form—whether of tools, emotions, or social interactions—are grounded in bodily experiences. Thus, cognition is inherently *situated*, shaped by the ways in which we physically engage with the world.

Such insights have practical applications in fields as diverse as psychotherapy, education, and rehabilitation. Somatic therapies, which leverage movement and body awareness, draw upon this embodied cognition framework to facilitate emotional regulation and trauma recovery. For example, sensorimotor psychotherapy emphasises the role of bodily sensations and movements in processing traumatic memories, arguing that unresolved trauma manifests as disruptions in the body's sensory-motor patterns.

Similarly, mindful movement practices such as Tai Chi or Feldenkrais enhance cognitive and emotional functioning by restoring harmony between mind and body, supporting the view that movement forms a foundational pillar of mental health.

Yet, it is important to recognise that the relationship between movement and cognition is neither simplistic nor unidirectional. Movement patterns are influenced by cultural norms, personal history, and psychological conditioning, which in turn shape cognitive and emotional outcomes. For instance, individuals habituated to restrained or inhibited movement may experience diminished emotional expressivity or awareness, underscoring how social context and individual biography modulate the embodied mind. Furthermore, pathological conditions such as Parkinson's disease, which impair motor function, often coincide with cognitive and affective difficulties, illustrating the integral nature of sensorimotor processes in psychological health.

This synthesis of neuroscience, psychology, and phenomenology challenges reductive understandings of cognition and highlights the necessity of reconceptualising the brain as part of a *sensorimotor system* rather than an isolated command centre. It invites professionals and scholars alike to reconsider how therapeutic interventions, educational models, and workplace designs might incorporate movement as a fundamental element of cognitive and emotional functioning. Recognising the embodied brain means acknowledging that thought, mood, and identity emerge through the ongoing dialogue between muscles and mind—a dialogue that is both profoundly personal and universally human.

As research deepens, it becomes increasingly clear that to neglect the body's role in cognition is to ignore a vital dimension of psychological life. The muscles do not merely carry us through space; they are active participants in shaping who we are and how we feel. This perspective not only broadens our understanding of the mind but opens pathways to richer, more integrated approaches to mental health and human potential. By embracing the embodied brain, we reclaim movement as a primary language of cognition—one that speaks as eloquently as words and thoughts, weaving together the threads of perception, emotion, and action into the fabric of lived experience.

Neural Rhythms, Physical Rhythms

Few phenomena illustrate the intimate connection between body and brain more vividly than rhythm. The steady beat of footsteps, the cadence of a dance, the pulsation of breath—all these physical rhythms do more than mark time; they resonate deeply within the brain's neural circuits, shaping cognition, emotion, and behaviour. To appreciate how rhythmic physical activity tunes the brain for mood regulation and problem-solving is to confront a profound aspect of human nature that has been obscured by reductionist models separating mind and body. Rhythmic movement is not merely a mechanical repetition but a dynamic synchronisation that entrains neural oscillations, fostering mental states conducive to clarity, creativity, and emotional balance.

At the heart of this synchrony lies the brain's inherent oscillatory activity—patterns of rhythmic electrical firing across networks of neurons. These neural oscillations, observed in various frequency bands such as alpha, beta, theta, and gamma waves, underpin essential cognitive functions including attention, memory encoding, and emotional regulation. Crucially, these brain rhythms are not static; they are modulated by sensory input and motor activity, reflecting a continuous dialogue between the internal neural milieu and external bodily movement. The relationship between physical rhythm and neural oscillations forms a feedback loop whereby the body's motion can entrain and stabilise brain rhythms, enhancing neural coherence and functional connectivity.

Consider walking, an activity so commonplace it often escapes notice, yet it offers a striking example of this embodied neural tuning. Neuroimaging studies demonstrate that the rhythmic pattern of gait influences brainwave synchronisation, particularly within networks linked to executive function and emotional regulation. Walking at a natural, steady pace engages sensorimotor regions alongside limbic structures implicated in mood, producing an alignment of neural oscillations that promotes mental stability and cognitive flexibility. This effect is not confined to solitary movement;

synchronized walking within groups amplifies these neural harmonisations, reinforcing social bonding and collective emotional states. The ancient human practice of communal walking or marching, therefore, can be understood as a profound neurological synchroniser as much as a social ritual.

Dancing extends this principle into more complex, multi-dimensional movement patterns, coupling rhythm with expressive gesture and social interaction. Studies in neuropsychology reveal that dance stimulates widespread neural networks, including motor, auditory, and prefrontal regions, fostering enhanced neuroplasticity and emotional regulation. The synchronisation required for coordinated dance movements engages the brain's mirror neuron system, enhancing empathy and social cognition. Moreover, rhythmic entrainment during dance has been linked to increased release of neurotransmitters such as dopamine and endorphins, chemicals central to reward processing and mood elevation. This neurochemical cascade provides a physiological basis for the well-documented mood-enhancing effects of dance, making it a potent modality for both individual and collective emotional health.

Yet the relationship between rhythm and brain function is not without complexity. While rhythmic entrainment generally supports cognitive and emotional resilience, disruptions in neural oscillations are implicated in a range of psychiatric and neurological disorders, including depression, schizophrenia, and Parkinson's disease. In these conditions, the brain's capacity to maintain stable rhythms is compromised, leading to cognitive fragmentation and emotional dysregulation. Intriguingly, rhythmic movement therapies—such as rhythmic auditory stimulation and movement-based interventions—have shown promise in restoring neural coherence and ameliorating symptoms. These findings underscore rhythm's dual role as both a marker of neural health and a potential therapeutic tool.

The cultural dimensions of rhythmic movement further illuminate its neural significance. Across societies, rhythmic physical activities—whether tribal dances, military drills, or religious ceremonies—serve as vehicles for synchronising bodies and minds, reinforcing group identity and collective emotion. Ethnographic research highlights how shared rhythm in movement fosters social cohesion through the alignment of neural and physiological states, an effect mediated by the coupling of motor and limbic systems. This interplay suggests that rhythm is foundational not only to individual mental states but also to the emergent properties of social life, linking neural oscillations to broader patterns of human connection.

On a philosophical level, recognising rhythm as a bridge between body and brain challenges reductionist notions that isolate cognition within the mind alone. Instead, it invites a more integrated understanding of human experience as inherently temporal and dynamic—an ongoing process of entrainment where brain, body, and environment resonate in synchrony. This perspective reorients questions of mental health and cognitive function toward practices that cultivate embodied rhythm, positioning movement not as ancillary to thought but as a primary architect of mental life.

Modern applications of this knowledge are increasingly evident. Mindfulness-based movement therapies, rhythmic exercise routines, and even technologies designed to stimulate neural entrainment through external rhythmic cues reflect a growing appreciation of rhythm's centrality to psychological well-being. For example, programmes utilising rhythmic walking or drumming have been employed to support cognitive rehabilitation in stroke survivors and individuals with dementia, demonstrating tangible improvements in attention, memory, and mood. Such interventions translate the abstract science of neural oscillations into embodied practices that enhance quality of life.

However, the integration of rhythmic movement into mental health paradigms faces challenges, not least the dominance of pharmacological and cognitive-behavioural approaches that often overlook embodied dimensions. A critical, ethical reflection on this tendency reveals a persistent cultural bias privileging the mind's abstract functions over the body's lived experience. Embracing rhythmic physical activity as a tool for mental health thus requires not only scientific validation but also a cultural shift toward valuing embodied knowing. This shift entails recognising movement as a fundamental form of cognitive and emotional engagement—one that has been marginalised in clinical and educational settings but holds immense transformative potential.

In sum, the coupling of neural rhythms with physical rhythms constitutes a vital mechanism by which the brain and body co-regulate mood and cognitive function. Through the entrainment fostered by activities such as walking and dancing, rhythmic movement shapes neural coherence, facilitates emotional balance, and enhances problem-solving capacity. This insight invites a reconsideration of how we approach mental health and cognition, urging the integration of embodied rhythm into therapeutic, educational, and social practices. As we deepen our understanding of this profound connection, we open pathways toward a more holistic psychology—one in which movement is recognised as an indispensable language of the mind.

Stillness is a Modern Invention

It is easy to assume that stillness—remaining motionless, pausing the body—has been a natural or timeless state of human existence. Yet, when examined through the lens of evolutionary history, stillness emerges as a striking anomaly rather than the norm. For millions of years, motion was central to human survival, cognition, and emotional regulation. Our bodies and brains evolved in environments where continual movement was not optional but essential, finely attuned to the demands of foraging, hunting, and social interaction. The emergence of industrial culture, with its sedentary work patterns and mechanised routines, represents a radical departure from this evolutionary blueprint. This shift has profound implications for mental health, contributing to what many researchers now describe as a crisis of disembodiment and psychological distress.

Human evolution is inseparable from motion. From the earliest hominins walking upright across the savannah to the complex migratory patterns of hunter-gatherer societies, movement was foundational to our development. Bipedalism itself reshaped the human brain, freeing the hands for tool use and enabling complex gestural communication. Studies of hunter-gatherer groups today reveal that individuals routinely cover between 10 and 20 kilometres per day, engaging in varied, purposeful physical activity that integrates sensory input with motor output. This constant interplay between body and environment forged neural architectures designed to process information in motion. Far from being a mere backdrop, movement shaped cognitive capacities such as spatial memory, problem-solving, and social coordination.

The brain's reliance on motion extends to emotional regulation. The physiological states induced by physical activity—altered heart rate, breath patterns, and muscle tension—are intricately linked to affective experience. Evolutionary pressures favoured organisms capable of modulating arousal and mood through movement, enabling adaptive responses to threats and opportunities. For instance, fleeing predators or chasing prey necessitated not only physical exertion but rapid shifts in attention and emotional tone. This coupling of motion and mood became embedded in the nervous system, forming a fundamental aspect of human psychology.

Against this backdrop, the modern phenomenon of stillness—prolonged periods of inactivity—stands out as a relatively recent and culturally specific invention. Industrialisation introduced new modes of labour characterised by extended sitting, repetitive tasks, and minimal physical engagement. The rise of office work, mechanised transport, and screen-based entertainment entrenched sedentary habits that were previously absent or rare in human experience. While some forms of stillness, such as meditation or rest, have deep historical roots and can support mental health, the enforced inactivity of modern life is qualitatively different. It is often passive, fragmented, and accompanied by overstimulation from digital devices, creating a dissonance between mind and body.

This dissonance contributes to the growing prevalence of mental health disorders, many of which correlate strongly with sedentary behaviour. Epidemiological studies link physical inactivity with increased risk of depression, anxiety, and cognitive decline. The physiological mechanisms are multifaceted: reduced aerobic capacity impairs neurogenesis; lack of movement disrupts circadian rhythms and hormonal balance; and diminished sensory-motor engagement weakens the brain's integrative functions. Psychologically, sedentary lifestyles can exacerbate feelings of isolation, rumination, and emotional blunting. The very bodily states that once supported adaptive mood regulation are undermined, leaving the individual vulnerable to dysregulation.

Critically, the problem is not merely the absence of movement but the *quality* and *context* of stillness imposed by industrial culture. Unlike intentional stillness practised in contemplative traditions—marked by embodied awareness and integration—modern stillness often involves passive immobilisation coupled with cognitive overload. Sitting for hours in front of screens, disconnected from natural rhythms and physical sensation, disrupts the embodied self. This form of stillness lacks the restorative properties of natural pauses and instead fosters fragmentation between mind and body. The result is a form of disembodiment that undermines psychological resilience.

Understanding stillness as a modern invention reframes how we approach mental health and wellbeing. It calls attention to the need for re-embodiment—reclaiming movement as a primary mode of cognition and emotional balance. This perspective challenges the dominant health paradigms that focus narrowly on exercise as physical fitness or weight management, advocating instead for movement as a vital psychological practice. Incorporating naturalistic movement patterns, rhythmic activity, and intentional pauses can restore the neural and physiological systems evolved for motion, supporting mental clarity and emotional integration.

Moreover, the cultural valuation of stillness reveals underlying tensions. Western ideals often equate stillness with discipline, control, and focus, while associating movement with chaos or distraction. This dichotomy obscures the nuanced roles both play in mental life. Evolution teaches that motion and rest are complementary states—each essential when appropriately timed and embodied. The challenge of modernity lies not in eliminating stillness but in reconfiguring it to align with our embodied nature, fostering practices that cultivate mindful presence rather than dissociative inertia.

Real-world examples highlight promising approaches. Traditional societies often embed movement and rest within daily rhythms that honour natural cycles, offering models for sustainable embodiment.

Contemporary innovations such as workplace movement breaks, somatic therapies, and embodied mindfulness practices seek to counteract sedentary patterns by reintegrating movement and stillness. These interventions recognise that restoring the dynamic interplay between motion and pause is crucial for psychological health.

The history of stillness, then, is not simply about physical inactivity but about a broader cultural and evolutionary disjunction. By tracing how motion was central to human functioning and how industrial culture disrupted that equilibrium, we gain critical insight into the roots of modern mental illness. This understanding compels us to rethink the conditions of mental wellbeing, emphasising the restoration of embodied rhythm as a foundation for cognitive and emotional flourishing. Stillness, far from being an innate human state, is a product of historical and social forces—one that must be consciously reimagined to serve rather than undermine our psychological integrity.

Micro-Movements, Macro-Emotions

The subtle dance of the body often speaks louder than words—especially when it comes to our emotions. Before we have the chance to consciously label what we feel, our bodies begin to communicate through tiny, often unconscious movements: a restless foot tapping beneath the table, a slight shift in posture, a fleeting gesture of the hands. These micro-movements, seemingly insignificant in isolation, form an intricate language that reveals the undercurrents of our emotional lives. Far from being trivial or random, they are deeply entwined with mood and affect, frequently preceding and shaping conscious emotional awareness. Understanding this connection opens a window into the embodied mind, demonstrating how physicality and feeling are inseparable and how the body often knows before the mind can catch up.

Research in psychology and neuroscience has increasingly illuminated the role of micro-movements as somatic markers—physical expressions that signal emotional states prior to or alongside conscious experience. Antonio Damasio's somatic marker hypothesis famously posits that bodily feedback guides decision-making and emotional processing, rooting cognition in visceral sensation. Extending this framework, the study of micro-movements reveals a nuanced layer of embodied communication where shifts in muscle tension, eye movement, or breathing patterns provide nonverbal cues to internal affective shifts. For instance, studies have shown that subtle facial microexpressions, which last only fractions of a second, betray concealed or emerging emotions such as anxiety, contempt, or joy before they are consciously recognised or verbalised. These involuntary signals serve as a biological barometer, offering critical information about an individual's emotional landscape.

Postural adjustments further illustrate this phenomenon. Research demonstrates that minor shifts in seating position—leaning forward slightly, crossing and uncrossing legs, tilting the head—often reflect fluctuating levels of engagement, discomfort, or cognitive effort. For example, in social interactions, participants unconsciously mirror each other's micro-movements, a process known as nonverbal synchrony, which fosters empathy and rapport. Conversely, a breakdown in this synchrony can signal relational discord or emotional disconnection. This subtle choreography of movement underscores that our emotional states are not only internally felt but also socially enacted and detected through these micro-signals.

From a clinical perspective, micro-movements offer valuable insights into emotional regulation and psychological wellbeing. Conditions such as anxiety and depression often manifest in distinct movement patterns: repetitive fidgeting, trembling fingers, or restless shifting may indicate heightened arousal or internal distress. Conversely, psychomotor retardation—slowed or reduced movement—is a hallmark of severe depressive states. These somatic signatures provide clinicians with observable markers that complement verbal reports, deepening diagnostic accuracy. Therapeutic approaches like somatic experiencing and body-oriented psychotherapy leverage awareness of micro-movements to access and modulate emotional states that might otherwise remain implicit or suppressed.

Intriguingly, micro-movements also play a pivotal role in self-regulation. Neuroscientific evidence suggests that subtle motor behaviours help modulate arousal and restore emotional equilibrium. For example, repetitive motions such as foot tapping or finger drumming may serve a calming function, aiding individuals in managing stress or anxiety. These behaviours engage neural circuits linked to sensorimotor integration and affect regulation, offering an embodied strategy for coping that precedes deliberate cognitive control. This challenges traditional views that regard such movements as mere nervous habits or distractions, reframing them as meaningful physiological processes intimately connected to emotional homeostasis.

In daily life, these micro-movements form a constant, though often unnoticed, backdrop to our conscious experience. The body's restless shifts, gestures, and postural nuances weave a nonverbal narrative that shapes interpersonal communication and self-awareness. The field of embodied cognition highlights how such motor behaviours influence not only how others perceive us but also how we come to understand our own emotional states. For example, deliberately adopting certain micro-movements—such as expansive hand gestures or open postures—can shift mood and cognitive outlook, demonstrating a bidirectional relationship where movement and emotion continuously inform each other.

This interplay becomes particularly salient in high-stakes or emotionally charged contexts. Public speaking, negotiation, or conflict situations reveal how micro-movements betray underlying tension or confidence before words are spoken. The ability to read and modulate these subtle cues can thus enhance emotional intelligence and social effectiveness. Training in body language and nonverbal communication often emphasises awareness of these small gestures as keys to decoding and influencing emotional dynamics. Yet, the ethical dimensions of such knowledge warrant careful reflection. The capacity to detect concealed emotions through micro-movements raises questions about privacy and consent, underscoring the need for responsible application within interpersonal and professional settings.

Moreover, cultural variations complicate the interpretation of micro-movements, as different societies encode and decode bodily signals in diverse ways. What counts as a sign of discomfort or engagement in one culture may have a different connotation elsewhere. This cultural specificity demands nuanced understanding and cautions against universalising interpretations of embodied emotion. It also highlights the adaptability of micro-movements as communicative tools shaped by social context, further illustrating how embodiment is inseparable from cultural embeddedness.

From a developmental standpoint, infants and children exhibit micro-movements as primary modes of emotional expression before acquiring verbal language. Early research in developmental psychology notes that subtle changes in muscle tone, facial twitching, or gaze shifts convey emotional states and intentions, serving as foundational components of early social interaction and attachment. These observations reinforce the notion that micro-movements constitute a primordial language of emotion, one that precedes and scaffolds later cognitive and linguistic capacities.

The profound link between micro-movements and macro-emotions challenges reductionist perspectives that locate emotion solely within discrete brain regions or cognitive appraisals. Instead, it calls for an integrative approach recognising emotion as a holistic, embodied phenomenon manifesting across multiple levels of organisation—from neuronal firing to whole-body movement. This framework expands the horizons of psychological theory and practice, inviting exploration of how subtle physicality shapes the architecture of feeling.

Engaging with the language of micro-movements enriches our capacity for emotional self-awareness and interpersonal attunement. Cultivating mindful attention to these small signals can enhance emotional intelligence, improve communication, and deepen psychological insight. Therapeutically, fostering sensitivity to embodied cues opens pathways for accessing emotions that resist verbal articulation, facilitating healing and integration.

Ultimately, recognising that *small movements can reveal vast emotional landscapes* redefines how we understand the mind-body relationship. It asserts that emotion is not hidden behind layers of cognition but emerges dynamically through the body's restless activity. By attending to the micro-expressions and motions that precede conscious awareness, we uncover a richer, more textured understanding of human emotion—one that honours the body's wisdom and expands the possibilities for psychological growth and connection.

Chapter 2
Feeling in Flesh

Emotion is so often imagined as something airy and abstract, a drama staged only in the mind—given shape through words, recollections, or conscious thought. But this tidy intellectual picture leaves out a more primal truth: feelings begin as bodily stirrings. They register first in pulse and breath, in the tightening of muscle or the slow drop of the stomach, long before they reach the threshold of language. Antonio Damasio's influential somatic marker hypothesis broke open this understanding by proposing that bodily feedback—accelerated heartbeat, shifts in hormone flow, subtle muscular contractions—functions as a compass in both decision-making and emotional awareness. Eugene Gendlin, too, with his notion of the "felt sense," gave language to the inarticulate bodily knowing that carries meaning before words can catch it. This chapter opens from those foundations, treating the body not as the stage upon which emotions appear but as their very birthplace.

From here, the terrain broadens to consider how moods leave their traces across the body's landscape. Somatic traditions have long understood this: Qi Gong's flowing gestures, the Alexander Technique's re-education of posture, or the embodied insights carried in yoga and martial arts—all recognise that emotions settle in sinew and bone, in the tissues themselves. Modern therapeutic practices echo this wisdom. Trauma work often reveals distress written into physical patterns—tightness in the chest, a lump caught at the throat, a dragging heaviness in the legs. These maps of mood are not poetic flourishes but evidence of a deep intertwining: physiology and emotion in ceaseless dialogue, each impressing itself upon the other.

Nowhere is this interconnection more evident than when feeling is denied expression or trauma goes unresolved. "When the body says no"—a phrase Gabor Maté has made indelible—captures the way unresolved conflict can reappear in the language of illness: chronic fatigue, unexplained pain, even autoimmune disorders. Symptoms such as these are not aberrations but somatic testimonies, the body speaking where the voice cannot. They unsettle the neat boundary between mind and matter, pressing us to acknowledge movement, touch, and embodied awareness as indispensable tools in restoring conversation within the self. By turning toward sensation rather than away from it, one begins to read these bodily messages and, in doing so, opens a path toward healing that attends to psyche and flesh alike.

The chapter also seeks to rescue movement from its narrow framing as exercise, correction, or bodily ornamentation. Here, movement becomes a practice of radical listening, a way of attuning to the body's quiet intelligence. It is less about sculpting or repairing and more about bearing witness—staying with the weight of an emotion as it courses through the chest, or noticing the tremor in a hand as a sign rather than a flaw. This turn from doing to attending shifts the axis entirely: movement as presence, as emotional literacy, as the ground from which resilience can grow.

What follows is a weaving of science, cultural tradition, and lived practice. The aim is neither reduction to pure biology nor abstraction into metaphor, but a fuller picture in which the flesh is understood as the very medium of feeling. To sense with the body is not secondary to thought—it is the foundation upon which thought rests. This chapter extends an invitation to recognise the body as co-author in the story of emotion, keeper of truths unspoken, and a partner in the work of healing and transformation.

Somatic Markers and the Felt Sense

The notion that emotion originates solely within the mind as a product of thought or language is a misconception that has long shaped psychological theory and popular understanding alike. Yet, emerging from the shadows of cognitive reductionism is a more nuanced and profoundly embodied perspective: emotion begins as a physical signal within the body, a visceral experience that precedes and informs conscious awareness and verbal expression. Two landmark frameworks illuminate this embodied genesis of feeling—Antonio Damasio's somatic marker hypothesis and Eugene Gendlin's concept of the "felt sense." Together, they challenge the primacy of abstract cognition by positing that bodily sensations constitute the raw material from which emotion and decision-making arise, anchoring psychological life firmly in the flesh.

Damasio's somatic marker hypothesis, introduced in the 1990s, represents a paradigm shift in neuroscience and affective science. At its core is the idea that bodily signals—changes in heart rate, hormonal shifts, muscle tension—act as "markers" that guide cognition and behaviour. These somatic markers arise from the body's interaction with its environment and are mapped onto brain circuits involved in emotion and decision-making, particularly within the ventromedial prefrontal cortex. Crucially, these bodily signals do not simply accompany emotional experience; they *shape* it, providing an embodied context that helps the brain evaluate choices rapidly and effectively. Patients with damage to this brain region, unable to generate or interpret somatic markers, exhibit profound deficits in decision-making despite intact intellectual faculties, underscoring the indispensable role of the body in emotional cognition.

The practical implications of somatic markers are manifold. Consider a scenario where an individual contemplates a risky business venture. Rather than relying purely on analytical calculation, the body generates subtle cues—an uneasy gut feeling, a tightening chest—that flag potential danger. These signals are often non-conscious yet guide the individual away from decisions that might lead to harm. Somatic markers thus function as an embodied heuristic, a shortcut that integrates past emotional learning and physiological feedback to inform present choices. This challenges the classic rationalist view of decision-making as detached and purely cerebral, highlighting instead how bodily experience is woven into the fabric of cognition.

Eugene Gendlin's concept of the "felt sense" complements and deepens this understanding by focusing on the pre-verbal, tacit bodily awareness that carries meaning beyond explicit thought. Gendlin, a philosopher and psychotherapist, observed that clients often struggle to articulate complex emotional states until they learn to attend to the vague, holistic sensation within the body that precedes language. This "felt sense" is neither purely physical nor purely mental; it is an integrated, bodily-felt meaning that encapsulates emotional, cognitive, and existential dimensions. It is a living, dynamic experience that can be accessed and explored through focused attention, often leading to profound insight and emotional resolution.

The felt sense thus functions as a bridge between embodied sensation and conscious understanding. It illustrates how emotion is not merely a byproduct of mental appraisal but a fundamental way in which the body "knows" and interprets experience. This has transformative consequences for therapy and self-awareness practices. For example, focusing on the felt sense allows individuals to engage with emotions that are diffuse or suppressed, fostering a deeper connection with their inner life. It reframes emotional awareness from a cognitive exercise into a somatic dialogue, emphasising *listening* to the body rather than analysing or suppressing feelings.

Both somatic markers and the felt sense reveal emotion as inherently embodied—a process beginning in the physical terrain of the body before ascending to the heights of thought and language. This insight challenges dualistic separations that have historically cast body and mind as distinct or hierarchical. Instead, emotion is revealed as a dynamic interplay, a continual feedback loop where bodily signals inform cognitive appraisal and cognition, in turn, modulates bodily response. This interaction is foundational not only to emotional experience but also to identity, motivation, and interpersonal connection.

Recent research continues to expand on these ideas, exploring how interoception—the brain's ability to sense internal bodily states—mediates emotional experience. Studies indicate that individuals with greater interoceptive awareness tend to exhibit more nuanced emotional regulation and empathy. Conversely, disruptions in this embodied awareness are implicated in psychiatric conditions such as anxiety, depression, and alexithymia, where the capacity to identify and describe emotions is impaired. Therapeutic approaches that cultivate somatic attunement—whether through mindfulness, body psychotherapy, or sensorimotor techniques—leverage the principles of somatic markers and felt sense to restore emotional integration and resilience.

This embodied framework also prompts reconsideration of how we understand language and cognition. Emotions often resist immediate verbalisation precisely because they are grounded in pre-linguistic bodily experience. The felt sense accounts for this liminal space where meaning is implicit, embodied but not yet articulated. Language emerges from this somatic substrate, shaped by but never fully capturing the richness of felt experience. Thus, emotional literacy involves cultivating sensitivity to bodily signals alongside verbal expression, enriching communication with oneself and others.

Critically, this perspective invites an ethical reflection on the cultural tendencies to privilege rationality and verbal reasoning over embodied knowing. Such biases risk alienating individuals from their somatic wisdom, perpetuating disembodiment and emotional fragmentation. Embracing somatic markers and the felt sense as central to emotional life challenges these hierarchies, calling for educational, clinical, and social practices that honour the body's role in shaping mind and feeling.

In everyday life, attuning to somatic markers and the felt sense can transform decision-making, emotional regulation, and self-understanding. It encourages a practice of *embodied attention*—noticing bodily signals without judgment, allowing them to inform rather than be overridden by habitual cognitive patterns. This stance cultivates a deeper trust in the body's intelligence, revealing how much of what we call emotion is first experienced beneath the threshold of conscious thought.

Ultimately, the insights of Damasio and Gendlin affirm that emotion is not an abstract mental category but a living, breathing interplay of body and brain. They demonstrate that feeling begins in flesh, that the body speaks a language of signals and sensations which the mind learns to interpret and embody. This embodied genesis of emotion redefines our understanding of the human psyche, offering a profound path toward integrating body, mind, and feeling into a coherent whole.

Mood Maps of the Body

Emotions are rarely confined to abstract mental states; they are profoundly somatic, lived experiences that register in the body's tissues, posture, and movement. Across cultures and healing traditions, there is a shared recognition that moods do not simply colour the mind but manifest palpably within the body—what one might call "living moods." This chapter's exploration of mood maps draws on this embodied understanding, weaving together insights from somatic practices such as Qi Gong, the Alexander Technique, and contemporary trauma-informed body mapping to demonstrate how different emotional states imprint themselves on physical experience. These practices reveal the body not as a neutral vessel but as a richly textured landscape where moods dwell, express, and inform.

Qi Gong, a millennia-old Chinese movement and meditation practice, offers a vivid illustration of mood's embodiment. Rooted in the concept of qi—the vital life force flowing through energy channels—Qi Gong emphasises the cultivation and regulation of bodily energy to harmonise mind and emotion. Practitioners learn to perceive how tension, stagnation, or imbalance in specific areas correspond to emotional blockages. For example, tightness in the chest might indicate grief or anxiety, while constricted movement in the hips may reflect suppressed anger or fear. Through slow, deliberate movements and breath awareness, Qi Gong guides the practitioner in restoring the flow of qi, which simultaneously alleviates physical discomfort and transforms emotional tone. The practice embodies the principle that moods inhabit the body's energy system and can be modulated through embodied attention.

Parallel insights arise in the Alexander Technique, a Western somatic education method developed in the early 20th century. Though primarily aimed at improving posture and movement efficiency, Alexander Technique also highlights the emotional narratives encoded in habitual bodily patterns. Practitioners observe how chronic tension in the neck and shoulders often corresponds with stress or emotional holding, while restricted breathing patterns may indicate underlying anxiety. The technique's core involves cultivating *inhibition*—a conscious pausing that interrupts automatic physical and emotional reactions—and *direction*, a mindful reorientation of the body that fosters ease and openness. By changing physical habits, individuals often report shifts in mood and emotional resilience, underscoring the inseparability of body and feeling. The Alexander Technique thus acts as a practical tool for re-mapping the body's emotional terrain.

More recently, trauma therapy has integrated body mapping to visualize and work with how emotional trauma imprints itself somatically. Trauma survivors frequently report that certain body areas "carry" the weight of past experiences—manifesting as chronic pain, numbness, or hypervigilance localized in muscles or connective tissue. Body mapping in therapy involves collaboratively identifying these somatic sites of distress and linking them to emotional narratives, offering a visual and experiential framework for healing. This process externalises internal experience, validating the body's role as an archive of mood and trauma. Studies indicate that such somatic approaches can reduce symptoms of PTSD and complex trauma by re-establishing communication between body and mind, allowing suppressed emotions to surface and integrate.

This culturally and clinically diverse evidence converges on a crucial insight: moods and emotions are not ethereal phenomena but embodied states with distinct physical signatures. They shape and are shaped by muscle tone, posture, breathing, and movement patterns. For instance, joy often manifests as an expansive chest and open gestures; sadness may present as a sinking of the torso and slowed movement; anger can be felt as heat and tension in the jaw or fists. These bodily patterns act as *mood maps*—spatial, sensory representations of affective states that offer a somatic vocabulary for feelings that sometimes elude verbal description.

The concept of mood maps invites a critical re-examination of how emotional experience is understood in psychological and medical paradigms. Conventional approaches frequently prioritise cognitive appraisal or neurochemical explanations while marginalising the somatic dimension. This can result in treatments that overlook the embodied substrate of emotion, limiting their efficacy. Integrating mood maps into therapeutic practice encourages a more holistic perspective, recognising the body's intelligence and its capacity to signal emotional states before the mind fully processes them. Such integration fosters deeper emotional awareness, self-regulation, and resilience.

However, engaging with mood maps also requires sensitivity to individual and cultural variation. The somatic expression of emotion is not universal; it is shaped by personal history, social conditioning, and cultural meaning. For example, the Western cultural ideal of controlled, upright posture may suppress overt bodily expressions of sadness or anger, whereas other cultures valorise expressive movement as a means of emotional release. This variability highlights the importance of contextualising mood maps within the lived realities of each person, avoiding reductive or one-size-fits-all interpretations. It also underscores the dynamic nature of embodied emotion, which is always situated within social and cultural frameworks.

Practically, attuning to mood maps can transform everyday life and therapeutic work. Cultivating embodied awareness through somatic practices enhances the ability to detect subtle bodily signals that indicate shifts in emotional state, allowing for timely regulation before escalation. This can improve interpersonal communication by making nonverbal cues more transparent and meaningful. Furthermore, movement modalities that engage the body's mood maps—such as dance therapy, somatic psychotherapy, or mindful movement—can facilitate emotional processing and integration, particularly for those whose trauma or emotional pain resists verbal articulation.

The richness of mood maps lies not only in their explanatory power but also in their invitation to *listen* deeply to the body's emotional language. This challenges the prevailing notion that emotions are primarily cognitive phenomena, repositioning them as fundamentally embodied experiences that demand an equally embodied approach to understanding and healing. By recognising that moods inhabit the body's landscape, we open new avenues for psychological insight, therapeutic innovation, and personal transformation. The body, with its intricate mood maps, becomes not only a repository of feeling but an active, intelligent partner in the unfolding of emotional life.

When the Body Says No

The body's language is often louder and more honest than the words we speak, particularly when it comes to emotions we have suppressed or trauma left unprocessed. The phrase "when the body says no," popularised by Dr Gabor Maté, encapsulates a profound truth that modern medicine and psychology are only beginning to fully appreciate: emotional repression and unresolved trauma do not merely reside in the psyche but find expression in physical ailments—ranging from chronic fatigue and fibromyalgia to autoimmune diseases and other systemic disorders. This somatic manifestation of psychological distress challenges the traditional mind-body divide and underscores the necessity of listening to the body as a vital source of information about emotional wellbeing. Moreover, it makes a compelling case that movement, far from being a peripheral activity, can serve as a crucial modality to restore the internal dialogue disrupted by emotional blockage.

The biological mechanisms linking suppressed emotion to physical illness have garnered increasing scientific validation. Chronic stress, often a byproduct of emotional suppression, triggers sustained activation of the hypothalamic-pituitary-adrenal (HPA) axis, leading to elevated cortisol levels and systemic inflammation. Over time, this physiological state undermines immune function, disrupts hormonal balance, and alters neural pathways involved in pain perception and mood regulation. The immune system, intricately intertwined with the nervous and endocrine systems, becomes dysregulated, giving rise to conditions such as rheumatoid arthritis, lupus, and multiple sclerosis. These diseases are not merely "physical" but embody the cumulative burden of unexpressed or unintegrated emotional experience. This biopsychosocial model reframes illness as an embodied narrative of lived psychological reality rather than a purely mechanistic malfunction.

Case studies illustrate this intimate connection. Patients with autoimmune disorders frequently report histories of trauma, chronic stress, or emotional neglect, often linked with patterns of emotional repression. For example, a woman diagnosed with systemic lupus erythematosus described years of suppressing anger and grief in order to conform to familial expectations, only to experience a sudden escalation of physical symptoms after a triggering emotional event. Such accounts are echoed in research demonstrating that adverse childhood experiences (ACEs) correlate strongly with adult onset of chronic illness, emphasizing that early emotional wounds imprint physiologically across the lifespan.

Trauma theory further elucidates how unprocessed emotional experiences become "frozen" in the body. Peter Levine's work in somatic experiencing highlights that trauma disrupts the natural completion of defensive responses—fight, flight, or freeze—leaving the nervous system in a state of dysregulation. The unresolved activation is stored somatically as chronic muscular tension, altered breathing patterns, or autonomic nervous system imbalance. This somatic residue impairs the individual's capacity for emotional regulation and often manifests as persistent physical symptoms, even when the original psychological triggers are not consciously recalled. Such understanding challenges psychotherapeutic paradigms focused solely on verbal processing, advocating for embodied interventions that access the body's stored memory.

Movement emerges as a powerful medium for restoring this disrupted internal dialogue. Unlike talk therapy, which primarily engages cognitive and linguistic faculties, movement re-engages sensorimotor pathways and physiological regulation. Practices such as yoga, dance therapy, and martial arts offer embodied modalities through which individuals can gently release chronic tension, increase bodily awareness, and re-establish flow in nervous system function. Neuroscientific studies support this: movement stimulates the vagus nerve, enhancing parasympathetic activity and promoting relaxation; it also increases neuroplasticity, aiding the integration of fragmented emotional experiences. Through movement, the body "speaks" what words may fail to express, allowing the person to reconnect with suppressed emotions in a safe, embodied context.

Importantly, movement for emotional restoration transcends the conventional fitness paradigm of exertion and performance. It is not about pushing the body to achieve external goals but about cultivating *radical internal attention*—a mindful listening to bodily sensations and impulses. This practice honours the body's intelligence and its subtle cues, fostering a compassionate presence that contrasts with the often judgmental or adversarial relationship many hold toward their physical selves. Movement becomes a form of somatic inquiry, a dialogue in which emotions are acknowledged and integrated rather than denied or overridden.

This embodied approach raises significant implications for healthcare and psychotherapy. Integrative models that combine somatic awareness with psychological support are gaining traction, recognising that healing requires addressing the whole person—body, mind, and emotion. Techniques such as sensorimotor psychotherapy, trauma-sensitive yoga, and somatic experiencing offer frameworks for clinicians to guide patients in re-establishing this internal communication. These methods acknowledge that the body's "no" is a vital signal demanding attention and response rather than dismissal or suppression.

Nevertheless, challenges persist in fully integrating these insights into mainstream practice. Biomedical models often marginalise somatic symptoms as secondary or psychosomatic, risking the minimisation of patients' lived experience. Cultural stigma around emotional expression further complicates individuals' willingness to engage with embodied therapies. Overcoming these barriers requires a cultural and institutional shift that validates the body's voice and promotes interdisciplinary collaboration between medical, psychological, and somatic fields.

For the individual, recognising when the body says no is an invitation to cultivate greater self-awareness and agency. It encourages attunement to physical sensations as valuable emotional data and fosters proactive engagement with movement-based practices tailored to personal needs. Such engagement can interrupt the cycle of suppression and somatisation, enabling emotional release and physiological restoration. Over time, this process supports resilience, emotional integration, and enhanced wellbeing.

Ultimately, the phenomenon of somatic illness as a manifestation of emotional suppression compels a rethinking of health and healing. It demands that we listen not only to what is spoken but to what the body reveals silently through pain, fatigue, and dysfunction. It affirms movement as a critical tool for re-establishing the internal conversation essential to psychological and physical health. When the body says no, it is speaking a truth that must be heard—and movement offers a pathway toward dialogue, understanding, and transformation.

Movement as Self-Awareness, Not Self-Improvement

In a culture fixated on optimisation, achievement, and aesthetic ideals, movement is too often reduced to a means of *improving* the body—sculpting muscles, burning calories, or enhancing athletic performance. This prevailing narrative frames exercise as a project of external transformation, where the body is an object to be fixed or enhanced according to socially constructed standards. Yet this instrumental view overlooks a far richer dimension of movement: its capacity to serve as a profound practice of *self-awareness*. When we shift our focus from changing the body to listening to it, movement becomes a radical act of internal attention—a dialogue with the lived experience of our flesh, sensation, and emotion that fosters psychological integration and authenticity.

The distinction between movement as self-improvement and movement as self-awareness is subtle but consequential. Self-improvement implies a goal-directed activity driven by external benchmarks—weight loss, strength gain, endurance—that positions the body as a site of achievement. This orientation can inadvertently cultivate alienation from the body, fostering a critical, objectifying gaze that disconnects the mover from their embodied experience. In contrast, movement as self-awareness invites a non-judgmental curiosity toward sensation, rhythm, and impulse, treating the body not as a tool for external ends but as a *source of knowledge* and presence. This form of movement prioritises *listening* over doing, *feeling* over controlling.

Historical and contemporary somatic practices exemplify this paradigm. The Feldenkrais Method, for instance, uses slow, exploratory movements to heighten proprioceptive awareness, enabling practitioners to discover habitual tension patterns and develop new, more functional movement strategies. This practice is not about pushing the body harder but about attuning to its subtle signals and reorganising movement with mindful attention. Similarly, the practice of Mindful Movement, rooted in contemplative traditions, emphasises embodied presence and sensory engagement as paths to psychological clarity and emotional balance. These approaches demonstrate that when movement becomes a practice of *internal dialogue*, it opens pathways to self-regulation, emotional insight, and resilience.

Neuroscientific research supports the transformative potential of movement as self-awareness. The brain's sensorimotor networks integrate sensory input with motor output in ways that shape not only physical coordination but emotional regulation and cognitive processing. Engaging in mindful, attentive movement enhances interoceptive awareness—the capacity to perceive internal bodily states—which correlates with improved emotional intelligence and reduced anxiety. This suggests that the benefits of movement extend beyond physical fitness, fostering neural plasticity that integrates body and mind. Movement, when approached as an embodied practice, cultivates a form of *radical internal attention* that rewires the brain for holistic wellbeing.

The cultural implications of reframing movement in this way are significant. In societies dominated by commodified fitness industries, movement is often co-opted into cycles of consumerism and perfectionism, where the body is disciplined through external regimes and quantified metrics. This can exacerbate disembodiment and shame, alienating individuals from their innate bodily wisdom. Embracing movement as self-awareness resists this commodification, reclaiming movement as an accessible, democratic practice rooted in lived experience rather than market values. It repositions the body as a *partner* in self-exploration rather than a project for external appraisal.

Importantly, this reorientation challenges the myth of movement as mere physical exertion. Movement as self-awareness includes stillness, gentle shifts, breath, and subtle postural changes—actions that may not register as exercise in conventional terms but are profound means of connecting with the body's emotional and sensory landscape. For example, slow, attentive stretching or spontaneous swaying can reveal tensions and emotions held beneath conscious awareness, facilitating integration. Such practices expand the definition of movement to encompass a continuum of embodied engagement that honours the body's complexity and nuance.

This perspective also has therapeutic resonance. Many psychotherapeutic approaches now incorporate somatic modalities recognising that trauma and emotional dysregulation are often stored in the body's habitual movement patterns and muscular holding. Movement as self-awareness offers a vehicle for accessing and transforming these somatic imprints. By cultivating a compassionate, present-centred awareness of bodily sensations, clients can reclaim agency over their embodied experience and foster emotional healing. This embodied approach complements verbal psychotherapy, enriching the therapeutic process with the wisdom of the body.

Everyday applications of movement as self-awareness invite individuals to shift from performance-oriented exercise to a practice of embodied curiosity. This might mean noticing the quality of one's breath during a walk, observing how different movements affect mood, or simply allowing the body to move spontaneously without agenda. Such practices nurture a sense of aliveness and presence that counters the fragmentation of contemporary life. They cultivate a *movement literacy* that extends beyond physical skills to include emotional and sensory fluency.

Reframing movement in this way invites a fundamental cultural shift: from viewing the body as a machine to be optimised, to recognising it as a living, sensing organism that holds vital knowledge. Movement becomes an act of listening, a dialogue with the self that honours complexity, vulnerability, and change. It calls on us to abandon reductive goals and embrace movement as a path to embodied knowing, where each step, stretch, or sway becomes an encounter with the aliveness within.

This transformation is not merely philosophical; it has practical urgency. In a world where disembodiment and emotional fragmentation are pervasive, cultivating movement as self-awareness offers a means to reclaim wholeness. It empowers individuals to inhabit their bodies with presence and compassion, dissolving barriers between mind and flesh. Through this radical internal attention, movement transcends its instrumental role and emerges as a vital language of self-understanding and psychological integration.

Chapter 3
Emotion in Motion

Emotion is so often spoken of as a force, yet to grasp its full nature we must see that it does not simply rise and fall in intensity—it carries direction. Feelings push and pull, they drag us down or send us surging forward, sometimes anchoring, sometimes lifting. Consider depression: it compresses posture, slows the body's pace, draws everything earthward. Anxiety, by contrast, propels—a restless forward lean, an energy that insists upon escape or action. To think of emotions as vectors rather than static states changes the conversation entirely. It frames them as dynamic energies, and movement—when entered into consciously—becomes a way of working with their momentum, not against it. In this light, the body ceases to be a mute container and becomes an active partner in navigating the emotional currents that shape our days.

Walking offers a particularly illuminating example. More than a method of getting from one place to another, it has long been regarded as ritual, as inquiry, even as a form of meditation. Virginia Woolf wrote of her reliance on walking to stir the creative process, to unbind thought and give emotions room to stretch. Nietzsche turned it into philosophy-in-motion, believing the deepest ideas come not at a desk but while striding through open space. In more recent memory, Steve Jobs conducted his now-famous walking meetings, swearing by the clarity and innovation the rhythm of footsteps seemed to summon. Across centuries, one sees the same principle at play: the gentle repetition of step after step steadies the body even as it stirs the mind, creating a synchrony in which reflection, regulation, and insight can flourish. Walking becomes both pilgrimage and therapy, a journey through the outer world that charts, at the same time, the inner.

Other traditions take the principle further into ecstatic release. Sufi whirling transforms rotation into prayer, a spiralling descent into states that dissolve selfhood and open towards transcendence. Meanwhile, the throbbing synchrony of rave culture—dismissed by some as mere indulgence—can also be read as contemporary catharsis: a collective ritual of sweat, rhythm, and vibration where unspoken feelings find voice through motion. In such spaces, movement does not tame or suppress the unruly force of emotion; it becomes its living embodiment. Through the body, chaos is enacted and released, and the darker intensities of human feeling are metabolised in the presence of others. What emerges is less performance than communal healing—a wordless conversation carried in the shared beat of feet and heart.

The entanglement of movement and feeling is so woven into human life that it saturates our language. We say we are "stuck," or that it is time to "move on." We talk of being "carried away," of "rising above," of "feeling weighed down." These phrases are not ornamental. Cognitive linguistics shows they arise from embodied frameworks: the brain organises emotions through sensorimotor experience, mapping feelings to directions, weights, and movements. Every metaphor betrays the body's imprint on thought. This constant borrowing of physical motion to articulate mood points us back to the deep circuitry that binds mind and flesh, reminding us that emotion is never purely mental—it is enacted, lived, moved.

Reframing emotion as motion carries profound implications for how we care for ourselves. Instead of trying to suppress or rigidly control feelings, one can learn to attend to their momentum: to notice whether a mood pushes outward, coils inward, or hangs suspended, and then respond through movement that allows that current to flow. Therapies rooted in dance, somatic practice, or mindful walking draw precisely on this principle. They invite people to reconnect with their bodies' signals and let the intelligence of motion guide integration. Healing, in this sense, is not about imposing order but aligning with the natural trajectories of feeling, learning how to ride them rather than resist.

This chapter follows these threads deliberately. It will trace how emotions move as momentum, linger over walking as a ritual of navigation, explore the ecstatic dances that court transcendence, and linger on the metaphors through which we understand affect itself. The hope is to reveal movement not as an adjunct to emotional life but as its medium—expression and regulation entwined.

The relevance is hardly abstract. Think of the writer pacing until an idea arrives, the pilgrim circling in devotion, the dancer in a club losing herself to rhythm, or the unconscious gestures—hands fidgeting, shoulders tightening—that betray moods we barely register. Each instance testifies to a truth: emotions live in motion. This chapter extends an invitation, not simply to think about that fact, but to inhabit it—to walk, whirl, sway, or pause with greater awareness of the momentum within, and to discover in that attentiveness new routes towards release, clarity, and a fuller sense of being alive.

Mood as Momentum

Emotions are not static snapshots; they are dynamic forces that propel us through experience, shaping not only what we feel but how we move and engage with the world. This concept—mood as momentum—posits that emotions carry directional energy, exerting physical and psychological pull or push that influences posture, movement, and behaviour. Depression, for example, often manifests as a downward, contracting force, heavy and grounding yet constraining, while anxiety projects a restless, forward thrust that can drive urgency and agitation. Understanding these directional vectors is critical because aligning movement with the natural momentum of our moods can facilitate emotional release, integration, and ultimately, psychological balance.

The idea that emotion has directionality challenges dominant models that treat affect as internal, isolated phenomena. Instead, mood is conceptualised as embodied momentum—an interplay of sensation, impulse, and action potential. Neuroscience provides support for this view, revealing how emotions modulate motor systems in the brain and shape habitual movement patterns. Studies of posture and gait, for instance, demonstrate that individuals experiencing sadness tend to adopt stooped, inwardly folded positions, while anxiety correlates with heightened muscle tension and readiness for rapid movement. These physical manifestations are not mere symptoms but part of the emotion's lived expression and regulatory feedback loop.

The implications for therapeutic practice and self-regulation are profound. By observing and consciously engaging with the directionality of mood, individuals can use movement to work *with* emotional momentum rather than against it. For example, rather than resisting the downward pull of depression by forcing upright posture in a rigid, superficial way, one might explore gentle, sustained movements that acknowledge heaviness while gradually inviting openness and lift. Conversely, the forward-driving energy of anxiety can be channelled into controlled, rhythmic movements that contain restlessness while allowing expression. Such attunement to mood's momentum fosters embodied emotional processing, reducing internal conflict and enhancing resilience.

Historical and cultural practices offer compelling examples of this principle. In traditional Chinese medicine and Qi Gong, emotional states are linked with specific bodily flows and directions. Grief is said to contract energy downward into the lungs, while anger rises through the liver and gallbladder meridians. Movement forms are designed to harmonise these flows, effectively "redirecting" emotional energy for balance. Similarly, somatic psychotherapies draw on the recognition that unresolved emotions become "stuck" in the body's kinetic patterns, and intentional movement aligned with these emotional vectors can unlock somatic blockages and restore flow.

Real-world applications further illustrate the efficacy of engaging mood as momentum. Consider the use of movement in depression treatment: interventions such as yoga and tai chi, which incorporate slow, mindful, expansive movements, can counteract the constricted, downward energy characteristic of depressive states. Studies show these practices reduce symptoms by improving mood and physiological markers of stress. For anxiety, practices that involve paced, repetitive motion—like walking or drumming—help regulate the nervous system by synchronising internal rhythms, providing a tangible outlet for forward-propelling tension.

This framework also reframes common experiences. The sensation of "feeling stuck" in sadness or "being pushed" by anxiety is not metaphorical but phenomenological, reflecting embodied momentum that has yet to find resolution. Recognising these forces invites compassionate curiosity rather than resistance, a willingness to explore how the body's movement patterns mirror emotional trajectories. This approach respects the inherent logic of mood, honouring it as a process rather than a problem to be suppressed.

Contrasting perspectives caution against oversimplifying the relationship between mood and movement. Not all emotional states fit neatly into directional categories, and cultural variations influence how emotion and movement are expressed and interpreted. Furthermore, some conditions, such as chronic depression or trauma, can disrupt the natural flow of emotional momentum, leading to stagnation or chaotic movement patterns. Therapeutic interventions must therefore be nuanced, adaptable, and attuned to individual complexity.

Nonetheless, the concept of mood as momentum opens fertile ground for integrating movement more deeply into emotional self-regulation. It moves beyond exercise as a prescription for health toward movement as an embodied dialogue with affective states. This reframing acknowledges the body's role in shaping emotional experience and offers practical strategies for harnessing movement's potential to foster healing and integration.

Ultimately, mood as momentum invites us to listen closely to the body's directional cues and to respond with movement that honours the flow of feeling. It reveals emotion not as a fixed state but as kinetic energy that courses through the body, shaping our posture, our gait, and our engagement with the world. By aligning with this momentum, we can transform the often burdensome weight of emotion into a dynamic process of release and renewal—an embodied conversation where movement and mood co-create the path toward emotional equilibrium.

The Walk as Ritual and Revolution

Walking is perhaps the most overlooked yet profoundly transformative act in the repertoire of human experience. Beyond its utilitarian function, walking has historically served as a deliberate practice of thought, emotion, and even rebellion. Far from a mere physical activity or exercise, it has been wielded by thinkers, artists, and visionaries as a tool for navigating the complexities of the inner world. The psychology of walking, as exemplified by figures like Virginia Woolf, Friedrich Nietzsche, and Steve Jobs, reveals an extraordinary capacity of this simple, rhythmic movement to catalyse cognitive breakthroughs and emotional processing. Through their varied but convergent uses of walking, we glimpse how motion becomes ritual and revolution—both a grounding ritual of presence and a radical movement of the mind.

Virginia Woolf famously described walking as integral to her creative process, noting that her best ideas often emerged during strolls through the streets of London. For Woolf, walking was a meditative practice that dissolved the barriers between inner reflection and external environment. Her ambles allowed for a loosening of mental constraints, inviting associative thought and emotional nuance. In her diaries and essays, Woolf links walking with the fluidity of consciousness, a bodily rhythm that mirrors the ebb and flow of ideas and moods. The act of walking here is not incidental but *constitutive* of her psychological landscape—a somatic scaffolding for creativity and emotional attunement.

Friedrich Nietzsche's relationship with walking was both philosophical and physical. Nietzsche walked extensively through the Alps, where movement through the natural world became a form of embodied contemplation. For Nietzsche, walking was a means to unsettle established thought patterns and

Dancing with the Dark

Dance is often celebrated as an expression of joy, celebration, or social bonding, yet beneath these familiar associations lies a more complex and profound dimension: dance as a conduit for confronting, processing, and integrating the darker facets of human emotion. Ecstatic and trance dance traditions—ranging from the spinning whirls of Sufi mystics to the pulsating rhythms of contemporary rave culture—embody movement as a form of collective emotional processing where catharsis takes precedence over control. This subchapter explores how such embodied practices create spaces for engaging with emotional depths often sidelined in everyday life, revealing movement's capacity to unlock, embody, and ultimately transform shadowed affective states.

At first glance, the ecstatic dances of Sufi whirling and rave culture appear worlds apart in form and context. Yet both enact a ritualised surrender to movement that transcends individual volition, inviting participants into altered states of consciousness characterised by dissolution of self-boundaries and immersion in communal rhythm. Sufi whirling, practiced by dervishes as a form of spiritual devotion, involves repetitive spinning that cultivates a trance state wherein dancers seek union with the divine. This spinning is neither frantic nor chaotic; it is a disciplined, intentional movement that channels emotional and spiritual yearning. The physical act becomes a vehicle through which ecstatic emotion is embodied and processed, allowing the dancer to move beyond the confines of ordinary selfhood and access a realm of sacred intensity.

Similarly, rave culture's dance floors pulse with hypnotic beats that facilitate trance-like states, collective effervescence, and emotional release. Despite being rooted in a secular, often hedonistic context, raves function as modern-day rites of passage where movement serves as a shared language for navigating complex emotional terrains—alienation, joy, grief, or transcendence. Here, dance is less about controlling the body's motion and more about yielding to the music's momentum, enabling the body to articulate emotions that defy linguistic capture. The communal aspect intensifies this process, as synchronized movement fosters a sense of belonging and collective catharsis, providing a therapeutic outlet for emotions suppressed in daily life.

From a psychological perspective, these ecstatic dance practices exemplify movement as a *cathartic process*, contrasting sharply with movement aimed at mastery or control. Catharsis, originating in ancient Greek tragedy, refers to the purging or purification of emotions, often through intense artistic or ritualistic engagement. Movement-based catharsis accesses pre-verbal, somatic layers of emotional experience that conventional talk therapies may overlook. Neuroscientific research into altered states induced by rhythmic movement supports this, showing that trance dance modulates neural circuits involved in emotion regulation, pain perception, and self-referential processing. Such states can facilitate emotional release, reduce anxiety, and foster integration of fragmented affect.

However, the cathartic function of ecstatic dance is not without complexity or controversy. The psychological concept of catharsis has faced critique for its simplistic assumptions that releasing pent-up emotion necessarily leads to healing. Some argue that cathartic experiences without integration can reinforce maladaptive patterns or emotional dysregulation. Yet, when contextualised within a structured, communal, and embodied practice, dance offers a container for safely navigating intense emotions, supporting gradual transformation rather than impulsive discharge. This underscores the importance of ritual and community in providing the holding environment necessary for catharsis to yield integration.

Movement as catharsis also engages with the cultural and social dimensions of emotional expression. Many ecstatic dance traditions arise within contexts where normative emotional expression is constrained or repressed. For example, Sufi whirling emerges from a mystical Islamic tradition that emphasises spiritual surrender amid social strictures, while rave culture often serves marginalized youth seeking alternative spaces for identity and emotional freedom. These practices create liminal spaces where socially taboo emotions—grief, anger, ecstasy—can be embodied and processed collectively. This challenges dominant cultural narratives that valorise emotional restraint and control, advocating instead for the recognition of movement as a vital mode of emotional truth-telling.

Ethically, the use of ecstatic and trance dance as emotional processing raises questions about consent, safety, and accessibility. The altered states invoked can leave participants vulnerable to psychological overwhelm or exploitation without appropriate support and boundaries. Contemporary practitioners and therapists integrating ecstatic dance into healing modalities emphasise the need for trauma-informed approaches that respect individual limits and provide grounding practices. This ethical framework situates movement as a potent but delicate tool for emotional work, necessitating skilled facilitation and communal care.

Practically, engaging with ecstatic and trance dance traditions offers individuals pathways to reconnect with embodied emotional intelligence. Such movement can disrupt habitual dissociation, reawaken suppressed affect, and foster a sense of aliveness often diminished in modern sedentary and cognitively dominated lifestyles. By embracing the chaotic, unpredictable, and even dark aspects of emotion through movement, participants cultivate resilience and a richer emotional repertoire. This somatic engagement deepens self-awareness, enriches relational capacities, and expands the scope of psychological healing beyond the verbal and cognitive domains.

Ultimately, *dancing with the dark* articulates a radical reimagining of movement as an active encounter with the full spectrum of human emotion. It recognises that healing and insight often emerge not through control or avoidance but through surrender and embodiment—through moving with the shadows rather than resisting them. This approach elevates movement from mere physical activity to a transformative practice of emotional reconciliation, collective catharsis, and spiritual exploration. In doing so, it affirms the body's indispensable role in navigating and integrating the complex, often ambivalent terrain of our emotional lives.

Motion as Metaphor

Language shapes thought, but the language of emotion is rarely abstract—it is deeply rooted in our bodily experience of movement. Expressions such as "moving on," "feeling stuck," or "being uplifted" are not mere figures of speech; they reveal a profound neurological entanglement between motor processes and affective states. This embodied metaphorical framework underscores that our understanding of emotion is inseparable from the ways we physically inhabit and move through space. Exploring motion as metaphor offers a unique lens to decode how the brain, body, and language coalesce, providing richer insight into the lived experience of mood and opening new avenues for emotional awareness and therapeutic practice.

The foundational idea that thought is grounded in sensory and motor systems is a hallmark of embodied cognition, a field that has transformed cognitive science over recent decades. George Lakoff and Mark Johnson's influential work on conceptual metaphors established that much of human thought is structured through bodily experience. For example, the metaphor "up is good" is nearly universal, linking positive emotions with upward movement—"feeling uplifted" or "high spirits"—and negative emotions with downward movement—"feeling down" or "low mood." These linguistic patterns reflect not arbitrary symbolism but fundamental sensorimotor mappings encoded in neural circuitry. Functional neuroimaging studies corroborate that processing metaphorical expressions related to movement activates motor and premotor areas of the brain, highlighting how language and embodied experience are intertwined at the neural level.

Consider the metaphor "moving on," frequently used to describe emotional recovery or progression beyond difficult experiences. This phrase captures the kinetic quality of emotional healing, suggesting that emotions have a vector—an impetus to shift forward through psychological space. The body's habitual forward motion during walking reinforces this metaphor, and experimental research shows that engaging in physical movement congruent with emotional metaphors can facilitate mood shifts. For example, walking forward after recalling a negative memory can promote emotional distancing and cognitive reframing, illustrating the bidirectional influence between movement and metaphorical thought.

Conversely, "feeling stuck" denotes an embodied sensation of immobility or blockage, often experienced in depression, grief, or trauma. This metaphorical expression aligns with the somatic experience of muscular tension, slowed movement, or postural collapse common in such states. Neuroscientific research into motor inhibition and affective disorders reveals that impaired motor initiation correlates with depressive symptoms, suggesting that the feeling of being stuck is not only metaphorical but grounded in motor system dysfunction. Therapeutic approaches that incorporate movement—such as dance therapy or somatic experiencing—seek to "unstick" the body, enabling emotional release and cognitive flexibility, thereby transforming metaphor into embodied practice.

The metaphor "uplifted" offers another vivid example of how motion encodes emotion. This expression encompasses not only the sensation of elevated mood but also physiological changes such as expanded posture, increased respiratory capacity, and lightness of movement. Positive emotions have been shown to broaden attentional scope and increase spontaneous gestures, reinforcing the upward, expansive qualities of uplifted mood. This interplay of language, body, and affect suggests that cultivating certain postures and movements can induce emotional states aligned with these metaphors, a principle employed in practices like power posing or embodied mindfulness.

However, the neurological and phenomenological entanglement of motion and metaphor is not always straightforward or universally consistent. Cultural variation shapes how movement metaphors are encoded and interpreted. For instance, some cultures may associate different spatial orientations with emotional valence, complicating the assumed universality of metaphors like "up is good." Moreover, individuals with motor impairments or atypical embodied experiences may engage with these metaphors differently, highlighting the need for nuanced understanding and inclusive application.

The ethical dimension of motion metaphors emerges in clinical and educational contexts. Recognising the embodied basis of emotional language challenges purely cognitive or verbal approaches to therapy and communication, advocating for embodied techniques that harness movement's metaphorical power. For example, encouraging clients to explore gestures or postures linked to metaphorical expressions can deepen emotional processing and insight. Yet, this must be approached with sensitivity to individual differences and cultural contexts, avoiding reductive interpretations or prescriptive movements.

Practically, integrating motion metaphors into everyday awareness enriches emotional literacy and self-regulation. Noticing how bodily sensations and movements align with metaphorical expressions provides a feedback loop that can inform mood management. For example, sensing a tendency to "feel stuck" might prompt intentional movement to stimulate flow, or adopting an "uplifted" posture might catalyse positive affect. Such embodied attentiveness cultivates a dynamic dialogue between body and mind, leveraging the power of metaphor to enhance wellbeing.

Ultimately, exploring motion as metaphor reveals that our emotional lives are not merely narrated by words but are *enacted* through the body's movement in space. This embodied linguistic architecture grounds abstract feeling in concrete physicality, bridging cognitive, affective, and somatic domains. By attending to the metaphors that shape how we talk about and experience emotion, we gain tools for deeper emotional awareness, richer interpersonal connection, and innovative approaches to psychological healing. Motion, then, is not only a physical phenomenon but a living metaphor—one that moves us, shapes us, and ultimately helps us understand ourselves.

Chapter 4
The Kinetic Self

We are accustomed to thinking of identity as something tucked neatly inside the mind—as beliefs, memories, or the stories we repeat to ourselves about who we are. Yet identity is not only housed in thought; it is lived through motion. The truth is stark: we do not merely *perform* movement patterns, we *become* them. Every habitual tilt of the head, every protective hunch of the shoulders, each unconscious rhythm of gait forms a choreography that quietly declares who we are. Beneath the surface of awareness, our bodies preserve and reveal our personal histories, our social masks, our most private sense of self. This chapter turns the gaze towards that kinetic dimension of identity, asking what it means to read the body as archive. At its centre lies Laban Movement Analysis (LMA), a framework that has, for over a century, provided language and structure for decoding the expressive content of human movement—a method widely employed in therapy, the arts, and somatic practice to touch what words often cannot.

Rudolf Laban's early twentieth-century system offers not a narrow technique but a robust vocabulary. It charts movement across four dimensions—body, effort, shape, and space—permitting a layered reading of gestures and patterns. A subtle tightening in the shoulders, the cadence of one's walk, the expansion of the ribcage: these details cease to be incidental and emerge instead as traces of inner life. Confidence may stride forward, fear may constrict, joy may lift. Through LMA we discover a provocative truth: identity is not fixed inside the mind but is continually enacted and reshaped through movement, always in flux, always in conversation with context.

Linked to this is the idea of posture as psychological record. How one "holds oneself" is more than a matter of bone and muscle—it is the cumulative script of lived experience. Years of shame may etch themselves into a collapsed chest and downward gaze, just as defiance may straighten the spine into rigid readiness. These are not mere reflections but active shapers of consciousness; posture both mirrors and reinforces emotional patterns, looping back into thought and mood. To study posture is therefore to encounter biography written in stance. The body remembers what the mind would prefer to forget.

This insight exposes the cultural obsession with *body image* for what it is: a narrowing of attention to surface appearance, crafted by societal ideals and external judgement. Against this fixation stands *body presence*, a far more intimate mode of relating to the self. Presence is not about how one appears to others but how one inhabits sensation—the felt aliveness of breath, weight, and movement. Where body image alienates, body presence reconciles, grounding identity in lived experience rather than projection. To cultivate it is to step out of the mirror and into the immediacy of one's flesh, an act that is both radical and restorative.

Yet the path is not straightforward. Many live in a state closer to inhibition than embodiment. Trauma, stress, or social conditioning can sever the dialogue between body and self, leaving us half-present, partly exiled from sensation. Practices such as yoga, martial arts, and somatic therapy strive to bridge that gap. Through rhythm, attention, and breath, they coax the individual back into the body, making it a home again rather than a battleground. They remind us that wholeness is not achieved by overriding the body but by listening—sometimes patiently, sometimes painfully—to its rhythms and messages.

The notion of identity as kinetic reverberates across multiple fields. Neuroscience, psychology, performance studies, even cultural theory—all find themselves challenged by the proposition that the body is not secondary but central in shaping who we are. This embodied lens resists reduction to narrative or cognition; it insists that movement, sensation, and psyche are entangled threads of a single weave. By embracing the kinetic self, one begins to see identity not as an inner possession but as a lived practice, always unfolding, always responsive.

The journey laid out in these pages invites readers into direct encounter with their own movements, postures, and bodily sensibilities—not as curiosities but as sources of genuine knowledge. With the guidance of Laban Movement Analysis and other embodied practices, we will trace how identity moves, stiffens, softens, and reforms. The aim is not correction or aesthetic refinement but recognition: to see the self not as a static form but as a kinetic process. In rejecting cultural scripts that equate the body with image, we reclaim it as a vibrant, expressive medium of becoming. The kinetic self, fluid and alive, is there for anyone willing to notice—to move through the world while simultaneously moving more deeply into themselves.

Identity as Movement Pattern

We are often inclined to think of identity as something fixed, a set of traits or narratives lodged within the mind. Yet identity is far more dynamic, continuously expressed and reshaped through the habitual patterns of our movement. This view proposes that we do not simply *have* movement patterns—we *are* them. Our habitual gestures, postures, and motor tendencies are woven deeply into the fabric of our selfhood, embodying the histories of our emotions, relationships, and social roles. To understand identity as movement pattern is to recognise the body as a living archive of who we are, and to appreciate how these patterns shape and reflect our psychological reality. This chapter draws on the rigorous framework of Laban Movement Analysis (LMA) to illuminate how movement encodes identity and how it can be employed in therapeutic and performance contexts to access and transform the kinetic self.

Rudolf Laban's contribution to movement theory transcends simple categorisation; he devised a comprehensive language for observing, describing, and interpreting movement that reveals the interplay of body, effort, shape, and spatial intent. LMA dissects movement into qualities such as weight, time, flow, and space, offering a multidimensional lens through which the complexity of embodied identity becomes visible. For instance, a person who habitually moves with sudden, bound efforts and contracted shape may be embodying underlying tension or guardedness, whereas fluid, expansive movements might express openness or emotional release. These movement signatures form a kinetic vocabulary that articulates unspoken narratives of selfhood, often more revealing than verbal accounts.

The practical applications of LMA have been profound, particularly in dance therapy and performance psychology. Dance therapists employ LMA to assess clients' movement patterns, identifying areas where emotional trauma or psychological rigidity manifests somatically. Through guided movement exploration, individuals can experiment with altering their habitual patterns—shifting from closed to open postures, modulating effort qualities—to foster emotional expression and integration. This process facilitates a reconnection with embodied feeling and offers a nonverbal pathway to self-awareness and healing. In performance psychology, LMA informs actors' and dancers' training by helping them embody diverse characters and emotional states authentically, demonstrating how movement shapes not only personal identity but also social roles and narratives.

Understanding identity as movement pattern also deepens our grasp of how early developmental experiences imprint on the body. From infancy, the ways we are held, moved, and responded to shape habitual neuromuscular patterns that become embodied templates for relating to the world. Attachment styles, cultural conditioning, and trauma all leave traces in these movement habits, influencing posture, gait, gesture, and expressive range. For example, a history of emotional neglect might manifest in constricted movement and limited affective expression, whereas secure attachment correlates with freer, more fluid movement patterns. Such somatic imprints underscore that identity is as much somatic memory as cognitive narrative.

Moreover, movement patterns are not static but evolve across the lifespan and in response to changing psychological landscapes. Identity as kinetic process emphasises plasticity and the possibility of transformation. Movement-based interventions that leverage LMA principles encourage experimentation and flexibility, inviting individuals to inhabit new movement patterns that expand emotional and relational capacities. This kinetic flexibility parallels psychological growth, underscoring the embodied nature of change. It challenges reductionist views that divorce mind and body, instead affirming a holistic understanding where shifting the body's habitual movement rewires not only motor circuits but emotional and cognitive frameworks.

Critically, recognising identity as movement pattern raises questions about agency and authenticity. To what extent are our habitual movements freely chosen versus conditioned by external pressures or internalised narratives? This tension invites ethical reflection on cultural norms and socialisation that shape bodily expression, often privileging conformity and control over spontaneity and presence. Dance and somatic practices informed by LMA offer spaces for reclaiming agency by exploring and expanding movement repertoires, enabling a more authentic and embodied self-expression beyond societal constraints.

Real-world examples underscore the potency of movement patterns in shaping identity. In clinical settings, individuals recovering from trauma frequently describe a sense of "learning to move again" as synonymous with reclaiming selfhood. Performance artists routinely engage with movement as a tool for inhabiting and communicating complex identities, using LMA's analytic vocabulary to craft nuanced physical narratives. Even everyday social interactions are suffused with movement-based cues—how we enter a room, greet others, or carry ourselves signals relational stances and internal states, continuously performing and negotiating identity.

This embodied perspective enriches the broader discourse on selfhood by situating identity not only in cognitive or linguistic domains but as a living, moving phenomenon. It calls for a recalibration of how we understand human experience, mental health, and creativity—inviting greater integration of somatic knowledge and practice. Identity as movement pattern is not a metaphor but a tangible, observable, and transformable reality that bridges mind, body, and social context.

As this chapter unfolds, readers will be introduced to the tools of Laban Movement Analysis and invited to reflect on their own movement patterns as mirrors of identity. Through this exploration, movement ceases to be incidental or secondary but emerges as a fundamental medium through which the self is enacted, understood, and evolved. The kinetic self is dynamic, expressive, and deeply revealing—waiting to be seen not only in how we move but in how movement moves through us.

Posture as a Psychological Archive

Posture is more than mere physical stance; it is a living record of our emotional history, social conditioning, and self-perception. How we "hold ourselves" physically encodes the weight of past pain, the imprint of cultural expectations, and the subtleties of our evolving self-image. This chapter delves into the profound ways posture functions as a psychological archive, storing layers of experience that influence not only our bodily alignment but also our emotional wellbeing and relational dynamics. Understanding posture as an embodied memory challenges the common perception of the body as a neutral vehicle, revealing instead its role as a dynamic site where psyche and soma converge.

Scientific inquiry into the body-mind connection has consistently demonstrated that posture and emotion are intimately linked. Classic research in psychophysiology reveals bidirectional influence: emotions shape posture, and posture modulates emotional states. A downward-turned head, rounded shoulders, and contracted chest often reflect and reinforce feelings of sadness or shame, while an erect spine and open chest can foster confidence and uplift mood. These postural patterns do not arise spontaneously; they are conditioned responses formed through cumulative experiences—traumatic or joyful—that leave lasting somatic traces. Posture becomes a nonverbal narrative of one's life history, a corporeal biography inscribed in muscle tone, skeletal alignment, and habitual tension.

The notion that posture archives psychological experience finds rich elaboration in the work of Wilhelm Reich and Alexander Lowen, pioneers of body psychotherapy. Reich identified "character armour" as chronic muscular tension that develops as a defensive response to emotional conflict and trauma. This armour shapes posture, restricting movement and expression, thereby maintaining psychological rigidity. Lowen extended this perspective by showing how posture embodies identity and emotional availability, advocating for therapeutic interventions that release somatic holding patterns to restore emotional fluidity. Such theories underscore that posture is not simply a physical attribute but a repository of unresolved emotional material.

Social roles and cultural narratives further sculpt our postural habits. Gender norms, professional expectations, and cultural ideals inform how individuals are taught to carry themselves—whether through upright, authoritative stances or modest, withdrawn poses. For example, women in many cultures are socialised to adopt closed, protective postures, reflecting and perpetuating societal expectations of demureness or vulnerability. These embodied social scripts become habitual, shaping the psychological landscape and influencing self-esteem and interpersonal engagement. Posture thus mediates the interface between personal identity and collective cultural forces, encoding relational and societal dynamics within the body.

Self-image, as internalised through both mirror feedback and interpersonal interaction, significantly informs posture. The way one perceives the body—its attractiveness, strength, or vulnerability—shapes how it is held and moved. Negative body image often correlates with collapsed, guarded posture, reinforcing feelings of insecurity or disconnection. Conversely, cultivating a positive, embodied self-image encourages postures that convey presence and openness. Practices such as the Alexander Technique, Feldenkrais Method, and somatic psychotherapy explicitly target postural re-education to align body and self-image, illustrating how modifying posture can recalibrate psychological experience.

Postural patterns also serve as early indicators of psychological distress or trauma. Chronic tension in specific areas—the neck, shoulders, lower back—frequently corresponds with emotional suppression or unresolved conflict. Psychosomatic medicine has long recognised these patterns, noting how posture and movement restrictions relate to conditions such as anxiety, depression, and PTSD. Emerging research in neurobiology reveals how trauma rewires sensorimotor circuits, resulting in persistent postural and movement alterations that embody the trauma's emotional imprint. This understanding informs therapeutic modalities that prioritise somatic awareness and postural realignment as pathways to healing.

The archival function of posture is not fixed or deterministic; it is a dynamic, evolving process responsive to intentional intervention. Through somatic practices and mindful movement, individuals can access and transform postural patterns, releasing held emotions and expanding expressive capacity. Such embodied work fosters greater self-awareness and emotional integration, allowing the body's psychological archive to be rewritten with new narratives of resilience and presence. This process highlights the plasticity of the kinetic self and the possibility of liberation from somatic constraints imposed by past experiences.

Ethical reflection arises when considering how posture is interpreted and addressed within clinical, educational, and social contexts. Misreading or pathologising postural expressions without attunement to cultural, individual, and situational nuances risks oversimplification and stigma. Respectful, empathetic engagement with posture as a psychological archive demands nuanced observation and collaborative exploration, honouring the person's embodied history and agency.

In daily life, posture continuously communicates our psychological state to ourselves and others, shaping relational encounters and self-perception. Becoming attuned to one's posture offers an accessible entry point to emotional awareness and self-care. Small shifts in posture can influence mood, cognitive clarity, and social presence, illustrating posture's powerful role in the embodiment of identity.

By viewing posture as a psychological archive, we expand the narrative of mind-body connection beyond metaphor into tangible somatic reality. The body emerges as a text inscribed with the layered stories of pain, joy, sociality, and selfhood—waiting to be read, understood, and, when necessary, rewritten. This embodied archive offers a profound resource for healing, growth, and authentic presence, bridging past and present through the living language of posture.

From Body Image to Body Presence

In a world saturated with images and ideals that equate worth with appearance, the concept of *body image* has become nearly synonymous with self-esteem, identity, and emotional wellbeing. Yet this fixation on how the body looks is not merely superficial; it carries profound psychological costs, fostering disconnection, self-judgment, and even pathology. To move beyond this culturally entrenched paradigm requires a radical reorientation—from an obsession with appearance toward cultivating *body presence*: an embodied state of aliveness characterised by deep sensory connection, attentiveness, and acceptance of the body as lived experience. This subchapter explores this crucial shift, arguing that true psychological integration and wellbeing arise not from how the body is perceived visually but from how it is experienced internally.

Body image, as traditionally understood, is a mental representation often shaped by social norms, media imagery, and interpersonal feedback. It is inherently comparative, evaluative, and frequently fraught with distortion. Studies reveal that dissatisfaction with body image correlates strongly with depression, anxiety, eating disorders, and diminished quality of life. These effects are amplified by the omnipresence of idealised body types in advertising and digital media, creating relentless pressure to conform to unattainable standards. Moreover, body image issues cut across gender, age, and culture, reflecting a global phenomenon that binds appearance to identity and social value. The cultural machinery that produces and sustains these ideals often does so at the expense of embodied authenticity and emotional health.

By contrast, *body presence* refers to an experiential mode of being grounded in sensory awareness and the felt sense of the body from within. It is less concerned with external appearance and more focused on the qualities of sensation, movement, breath, and proprioception—the sense of one's body in space. This shift reframes the body as a living organism with intelligence and agency rather than a static object for appraisal. Cultivating body presence involves practices that invite curiosity and acceptance, such as mindfulness, somatic therapy, yoga, and dance, which encourage participants to inhabit their bodies fully and without judgment. Research in psychology and neuroscience increasingly supports the benefits of such embodied awareness, linking it with improved emotion regulation, reduced stress, and greater self-compassion.

This transition from body image to body presence challenges prevailing cultural narratives that equate beauty with worth and promotes a more inclusive, compassionate framework. It recognises that focusing on appearance often obscures the richness of embodied experience and can perpetuate cycles of shame and alienation. Body presence, by contrast, fosters connection—not only to one's own sensations and emotions but also to others and the environment—thus supporting relational depth and resilience. It nurtures a form of *embodied selfhood* where identity is grounded in felt experience rather than external validation.

The therapeutic implications are significant. Interventions that prioritise body presence offer alternatives to cognitive-based approaches that may inadvertently reinforce disembodiment by focusing solely on thought patterns or verbal narratives. Somatic therapies leverage the body's capacity to store and express emotional truths, facilitating healing through movement, breath, and touch. For example, trauma-informed yoga and sensorimotor psychotherapy guide individuals to reclaim bodily presence disrupted by adverse experiences, enabling a re-integration of self that transcends distorted body image. These modalities underscore the transformative power of re-engaging with the body's felt reality as a path to psychological restoration.

Educational and social frameworks also stand to benefit from this paradigm shift. Incorporating body presence into curricula, wellness programs, and community initiatives can counteract the pervasive cultural emphasis on appearance. By fostering sensory literacy and embodied self-awareness from an early age, individuals can develop healthier relationships with their bodies and emotions, reducing vulnerability to body dissatisfaction and its sequelae. Such approaches promote holistic wellbeing, recognising the inseparability of body, mind, and social context.

Yet, embracing body presence does not deny the reality of societal pressures or the desire for physical self-care; rather, it situates these within a broader, more integrated understanding of embodiment. This perspective invites a critical stance toward cultural norms and encourages active resistance to commodified, appearance-driven ideals. It calls for creating spaces—both personal and collective—where bodies are honoured for their vitality and expressive capacity, not merely their conformity to aesthetic standards.

Practically, cultivating body presence involves cultivating *embodied attention*—the ability to tune into bodily sensations with openness and curiosity. This might mean noticing the flow of breath, the weight of limbs, or the texture of movement. Such practices nurture interoception and proprioception, foundational capacities for emotional intelligence and self-regulation. Through this attentive embodiment, individuals reconnect with the immediacy of their lived experience, fostering presence that enriches mental clarity, emotional depth, and relational attunement.

In shifting the focus from body image to body presence, we reclaim the body as a source of aliveness and meaning rather than anxiety and objectification. This transformation holds promise not only for individual healing but also for cultural change, challenging pervasive narratives that commodify and fragment the body. By prioritising inner sensory connection, we affirm a vision of embodiment that honours complexity, vulnerability, and vitality—a foundation for authentic selfhood and psychological integration.

This chapter will guide readers through this conceptual and practical terrain, offering insights and tools to embrace body presence as a radical alternative to appearance-driven selfhood. It invites a reimagining of what it means to inhabit a body—to move beyond looking *at* the body to living *in* it, fully and attentively. This embodied aliveness is not an abstract ideal but a tangible, accessible reality that holds the key to deeper emotional wellbeing and a richer experience of self.

Inhabiting vs. Inhibiting the Body

To inhabit one's body fully is to live with presence, attentiveness, and a fluent connection between sensation, movement, and self-awareness. Conversely, inhibiting the body signals disconnection, fragmentation, or dissociation—states that sever the natural dialogue between mind and soma, often as a protective response to trauma, stress, or emotional overwhelm. This subchapter contrasts these polarities—embodiment and inhibition—illuminating how inhabiting the body fosters psychological integration, while inhibition reflects disembodiment. Through examination of contemporary therapeutic practices and poignant survivor narratives, it offers compelling evidence and practical strategies for bridging this divide, underscoring the body's central role in healing and self-reclamation.

Embodiment, broadly defined, refers to the lived experience of inhabiting the body as an integrated whole—a dynamic interplay of sensation, movement, cognition, and emotion that grounds selfhood in physical presence. It involves *radical internal attention*, a mindful engagement with bodily sensations as sources of information and meaning rather than mere background or distraction. Neuroscientific studies highlight how embodiment activates interoceptive and proprioceptive neural pathways, enhancing emotional regulation, attentional focus, and resilience. This embodied state contrasts sharply with inhibition, where the body is partially or fully "shut down" in response to overwhelming stimuli or trauma, leading to numbing, dissociation, or fragmented experience.

Dissociation, as a form of inhibition, is a complex psychophysiological process often rooted in trauma. It serves as a survival mechanism allowing individuals to distance themselves from unbearable emotional or physical pain by detaching from bodily sensation or conscious awareness. However, prolonged dissociation impairs the integration of experience, leaving the individual disconnected from their own body and emotions. Symptoms can range from subtle emotional numbness and "spacing out" to profound amnesia or identity fragmentation. The body becomes a site of absence rather than presence, and habitual inhibition manifests as tension, rigidity, or paradoxical collapse.

Stories from trauma survivors vividly illustrate this dichotomy. Many recount an initial experience of fragmentation—feeling trapped in a body that no longer feels like their own, alienated from sensation and movement. Yet, through somatic therapies such as trauma-sensitive yoga, martial arts, or dance, survivors often describe a gradual *return* to the body, a reclaiming of presence that restores agency and emotional coherence. These embodied practices provide structured frameworks for safely engaging with bodily sensation, movement, and breath, helping to dismantle inhibition and foster inhabitation. For example, martial arts training cultivates mindful, intentional movement that builds strength, spatial awareness, and confidence—qualities that counteract the disempowerment of dissociation. Similarly, trauma-informed yoga emphasises slow, gentle engagement with sensation and breath regulation, offering a container for nervous system regulation and somatic reconnection.

The therapeutic value of inhabiting the body lies in its capacity to reinstate *embodied selfhood*, where the body is not merely an object but a lived, subjective experience. Embodied therapies leverage neuroplasticity, facilitating new sensorimotor patterns that integrate previously dissociated material. Clinical evidence shows improvements in PTSD symptoms, anxiety, and depression following somatic interventions, highlighting embodiment's role in emotional and psychological healing. This somatic integration supports greater emotional flexibility, groundedness, and a coherent sense of self.

Yet, the path from inhibition to inhabitation is neither linear nor universal. Some individuals may experience resistance or overwhelm when re-engaging with the body, particularly when prior trauma is deeply embedded in somatic memory. Ethical therapeutic practice requires attuned pacing, safety, and empowerment, respecting each person's unique readiness and boundaries. This cautious, client-centred approach underscores that inhabiting the body is a process of gradual reclamation, not forced confrontation.

Beyond therapy, cultivating embodiment offers profound benefits for everyday life. Practices such as mindfulness meditation, tai chi, or simple breath awareness cultivate moment-to-moment presence, enhancing sensory clarity and emotional attunement. These accessible tools empower individuals to notice early signs of inhibition—such as muscular tension or shallow breathing—and consciously shift toward inhabitation. Such embodied attention nurtures resilience, emotional regulation, and relational capacity, enriching psychological wellbeing.

Culturally, Western societies often privilege cognitive over somatic modes of knowing, fostering disembodiment through intellectualisation and suppression of bodily experience. The stigma surrounding emotional expression and bodily vulnerability compounds inhibition, isolating individuals from the richness of embodied selfhood. Challenging these cultural patterns calls for integrating somatic wisdom into education, healthcare, and community life, normalising body awareness as foundational to mental health.

Inhabiting versus inhibiting the body thus represents a fundamental axis of human experience, reflecting the degree to which we live integrated, embodied lives versus fragmented, disembodied ones. Reclaiming bodily presence is not simply about physical health but about restoring the unity of mind, body, and emotion that constitutes the whole self. Through mindful movement, somatic therapies, and cultural transformation, it is possible to bridge the gap—moving from inhibition born of pain and protection toward inhabitation marked by aliveness, connection, and psychological wholeness. This embodied reconnection is a radical, essential act of self-care and liberation.

Chapter 5
Exercise as Expression

Step into almost any modern gym and the scene feels familiar: walls lined with mirrors reflecting chiselled physiques, rows of machines promising sculpted precision, and an atmosphere charged with discipline—or, depending on your vantage point, vanity. Yet beneath this glossy surface lies something rarely acknowledged: the potential for these spaces to serve as ritual grounds, places where movement transforms into an act of expression, reflection, and, at times, transcendence. If approached with intention, the gym can cease to be a site of mere conditioning and become instead a theatre in which body, mind, and spirit meet in restless dialogue. The chapter you now enter proposes exactly this: exercise not as a relentless project of correction but as a practice of tuning into vitality, creativity, and emotional current.

The first pivot in perspective comes with distinguishing *training* from *tuning*. Training, in its conventional sense, presumes deficiency. It demands correction, improvement, sculpting, all governed by metrics imposed from outside. The body is treated as an instrument to be mastered, optimised, often coerced into compliance. Tuning, by contrast, imagines a different relationship: one of listening and responsiveness. Surfers speak of "reading the wave" rather than subduing it; fighters in the ring describe their bouts as dialogues of energy; dancers move in that delicate place between intention and impulse. Here movement ceases to be imposed and becomes instead a co-creation between body and circumstance.

This idea finds kinship with Mihaly Csikszentmihalyi's notion of *flow*, that elusive state where challenge and skill find balance, time bends, and self-consciousness slips away. Movement, in such moments, is neither obligation nor chore. It is joy—spontaneous, immersive, alive. Children remind us of this effortlessly: their games are unmeasured, unprogrammed, yet rich in developmental and emotional significance. But adulthood tends to strip play of legitimacy, branding it trivial, indulgent, unproductive. To weave play and flow back into exercise is therefore not escapism but reclamation: a necessary act for psychological vitality and creative flourishing.

Of course, such ideas clash with the realities of the fitness industry, which thrives on commodification. Movement, within capitalist logics, becomes product and spectacle. The industry sells us routines, bodies, equipment, identities, each bound to consumption. In the process, exercise risks being flattened into numbers on a machine or aesthetics in a mirror, its innate pleasures obscured. To resist this trend is to defend movement as something democratic, unpurchasable, a birthright of being alive. Exercise, thus reclaimed, belongs to everyone and owes nothing to consumerist ideals.

Examples exist all around if we care to notice them. Street dancers turn pavements into temporary sanctuaries of self-expression. Surfers, surrendered to shifting tides, model presence through rhythm and balance. Martial artists demonstrate that even combat can become fluid dialogue. In each case, what unfolds is more than technique or strength—it is ritual. These practices remind us that gyms, parks, dojos, even city streets can be consecrated as sites of transformation where movement is not merely action but ceremony, communication, communion.

The journey of this chapter will weave these threads together, examining how we might reimagine exercise not as drudgery or vanity project but as a layered art of inhabiting the body. We will look at what it means to practise *tuning* rather than *training*, to embrace joy and flow as serious modes of growth, and to resist the reduction of movement into yet another commodity.

Ultimately, readers are invited to rethink their own relationships with exercise—to regard each movement as an opportunity for presence, as dialogue rather than command, as artistry rather than obligation. To work out, in this light, is to discover the body not as object to be controlled but as companion to be engaged. Reframed this way, movement ceases to be a task. It becomes experience: textured, expressive, alive with meaning.

The Gym as Modern Ritual Space

Gyms, in popular imagination, are often dismissed as arenas of vanity, arenas where appearance is obsessively policed and bodies are sculpted in the pursuit of cultural ideals. This narrow view obscures a deeper, more transformative potential intrinsic to the space of the gym. When approached with intention, the gym can be reimagined as a modern ritual space—an arena where movement transcends mere exercise to become a deliberate act of self-expression, discipline, and psychological transformation. These spaces, often utilitarian in design and function, hold the capacity to serve as contemporary temples of transformation, where ritualised movement practices foster embodied presence, emotional integration, and identity renewal.

Ritual is commonly understood as a structured, symbolic practice that connects the individual to something larger—be it community, spirit, or a deeper self. While ancient rituals were often marked by sacred spaces and ceremonies, the modern gym offers a secular but potent arena where ritualised practices unfold daily. The repetition of sets, the deliberate pacing of breath, the focused attention on muscular engagement—all these elements constitute a kind of embodied ceremony. The gym's architecture and culture, with its dedicated zones, equipment arrays, and shared rhythms, create a physical and social container conducive to transformation. This container, when consciously engaged, facilitates a shift from distracted living into embodied presence.

Approaching the gym as a ritual space demands a reorientation of mindset and intention. Rather than a site solely for the correction or manipulation of the body, it becomes a place for dialogue with the self through movement. This reframing invites participants to cultivate *presence*—to inhabit the body fully in each repetition, each breath, each moment of strain and release. Such presence echoes the ancient concept of *praxis*, the unity of theory and action, where physical exertion embodies psychological and spiritual engagement. It is this ritualised embodiment that elevates gym practice from routine to transformation.

Real-world examples illustrate this ritual potential. Consider the weightlifter who approaches each lift with meditative focus, ritualising the preparation, breath, and execution as an act of reverence toward their body's power and limits. Similarly, group fitness classes often generate collective rhythms and shared intention, creating communal rituals that reinforce social bonds and mutual support. Even solitary runners describe the repetitive cadence of their movement as a form of moving meditation, a personal rite that integrates mind and body. These diverse practices demonstrate that ritualised exercise fosters a profound engagement with aliveness beyond the mere physical.

The psychological benefits of ritualised movement in the gym extend beyond immediate fitness outcomes. Ritual practices have long been recognised for their capacity to regulate emotion, reduce anxiety, and foster a sense of control and meaning. Neuroscientific studies suggest that the predictability and symbolism inherent in ritual engage neural circuits associated with safety and reward, creating conditions conducive to psychological integration. When gym routines are approached as rituals, they can evoke these neuropsychological benefits, transforming movement into a source of emotional resilience and psychological coherence.

Yet, tensions arise when the gym's ritual potential is co-opted by consumerist and performance-driven ideologies. The cultural imperative to commodify fitness often reduces gym practice to a transactional activity—paying for results, adhering to programmes promising efficiency, and measuring worth through visible outcomes. This commodification risks transforming ritual into mechanistic routine, eroding the embodied presence and symbolic richness that confer transformative power. Navigating this tension requires intentionality—a conscious reclaiming of the gym as a space for authentic engagement rather than performance spectacle.

Ethically, reframing the gym as a ritual space invites inclusivity and respect for diverse bodies and experiences. Ritual by nature is communal and connective; thus, gyms oriented toward ritual expression cultivate environments that honour embodiment in all its forms, countering exclusionary practices based on appearance, ability, or identity. This ethical stance aligns with emerging movements advocating for body-positive and trauma-informed fitness cultures that prioritise psychological safety and holistic wellbeing.

From a cultural perspective, the gym as modern ritual space reflects broader shifts in how contemporary societies seek meaning and connection amid fragmentation and digital saturation. Ritualised movement offers a tangible, embodied antidote to disembodiment, inviting participants to reclaim agency over their bodies and psyches. It reconnects individuals with the primal human experience of rhythm, breath, effort, and release, fostering a sense of rootedness and vitality often lost in modern life.

Practically, embracing the gym as a ritual space encourages new modalities of practice. Mindful movement techniques, breath-centred training, and community-oriented classes exemplify how gyms can support ritual embodiment. Trainers and practitioners who cultivate awareness of intention, presence, and symbolic meaning transform routine exercise into acts of personal and collective significance.

Ultimately, seeing the gym as a modern temple of transformation challenges prevailing narratives of fitness as vanity or obligation. It invites a radical reimagination of movement as ritualised expression—an embodied art form that integrates body, mind, and spirit. This perspective opens rich possibilities for psychological healing, creative exploration, and authentic selfhood, making the gym not only a place for physical change but a crucible for holistic transformation.

Training vs. Tuning

The prevailing paradigm in fitness and physical conditioning often frames movement as a process of *training*—a systematic effort to fix, improve, or control the body according to predefined goals and standards. Training carries connotations of mastery, discipline, and performance, emphasising outcomes such as strength, speed, or appearance. While this approach has undeniable benefits, it also risks reducing the body to an object of manipulation, fostering a relationship characterised by domination rather than dialogue. In contrast, the concept of *tuning* invites a more nuanced, responsive, and respectful engagement with the body, one that treats movement as an ongoing conversation rather than a conquest. This subchapter explores this fundamental distinction, drawing on insights from surfers, boxers, dancers, and somatic practitioners who describe their embodied practice as an art of attunement—listening to the body's rhythms, needs, and limits—and not simply a task to be conquered.

Training is often goal-oriented, rooted in a mechanistic model where the body is viewed as a machine to be optimised. It involves repetitive drills, quantified metrics, and prescriptive regimens designed to overcome perceived deficiencies or reach performance benchmarks. This approach has its origins in military and industrial efficiency models and has been amplified by modern sports science and commercial fitness culture. While effective for skill acquisition and physical development, training can engender disconnection from the body's intrinsic intelligence. It privileges external standards over internal sensation, potentially leading to strain, burnout, or injury when the body's signals are overridden or ignored.

Tuning, by contrast, emphasises sensitivity to the body's current state and an adaptive approach to movement. It is characterised by a *dialogical* rather than a *directive* relationship, where the practitioner continuously observes, feels, and adjusts according to internal cues. This mode honours variability, recognising that bodies fluctuate in capacity and readiness due to factors such as fatigue, emotion, or environment. Tuning prioritises embodiment and presence, cultivating a fluid interplay between intention and sensation that fosters both performance and wellbeing.

Surfers exemplify tuning as a way of being with the body and environment. They describe their practice as a dialogue with the ocean—reading the waves, adjusting posture, and timing movement in response to ever-changing conditions. This responsive, embodied attunement enables them to ride with grace and adaptability, embodying flow rather than brute force. The surfer's relationship with their body is one of partnership, where control is balanced by surrender to external forces and internal feedback.

Similarly, boxers cultivate a finely tuned awareness of their own bodies and those of their opponents. The sport demands not only strength and technique but also acute sensitivity to shifts in weight, rhythm, and intention. Fighters often speak of a "dance" or "conversation" within the ring, emphasising responsiveness over rigid domination. This attunement allows for strategic adaptation and preserves resilience by avoiding unnecessary muscular tension or injury. Here, tuning is integral to both effectiveness and longevity in practice.

Dancers, perhaps more than any other practitioners, inhabit the tension between training and tuning. Classical ballet, for example, requires rigorous training to master technique and achieve aesthetic ideals. Yet accomplished dancers also learn to tune into their bodies' subtleties—the quality of movement, breath, and emotional expression—to bring artistry and authenticity to performance. This tuning transforms movement from mechanical repetition into expressive embodiment, illustrating how disciplined training and responsive tuning coexist and enrich one another.

The distinction between training and tuning also has profound implications for psychological wellbeing. Training oriented primarily toward external outcomes can provoke anxiety, perfectionism, and alienation from the body. In contrast, tuning fosters a compassionate and curious relationship with oneself, enhancing interoceptive awareness and emotional regulation. Somatic therapists employ tuning principles to guide clients in sensing bodily signals and adjusting movement in ways that promote healing and integration, contrasting sharply with fitness models that prioritise exertion over attunement.

Technological advances in sports science and wearable devices offer new opportunities to bridge training and tuning. Real-time biofeedback, motion analysis, and heart rate variability monitoring provide objective data that, when interpreted mindfully, can enhance attunement to physiological states. These tools invite practitioners to engage in informed tuning—using external metrics not as absolute goals but as guides in an ongoing dialogue with their bodies. However, the risk remains that data become another source of control rather than connection, underscoring the need for embodied wisdom alongside technological assistance.

Culturally, the valorisation of training reflects broader societal values of control, productivity, and measurable achievement. Shifting toward tuning challenges these narratives by reclaiming movement as a lived experience that honours variability, vulnerability, and relationality. It disrupts binary thinking that equates success with domination and failure with weakness, instead fostering a spectrum where responsiveness and self-care are central. This paradigm shift invites a more inclusive and humane approach to movement, accessible across abilities, ages, and backgrounds.

In daily practice, tuning can be cultivated through simple but powerful habits: pausing to notice breath and sensation before movement, exploring subtle shifts in posture or rhythm, and embracing curiosity about what the body needs moment to moment. This mindful approach transforms routine exercise into a creative and compassionate practice, enhancing not only physical capacity but also emotional intelligence and presence.

Ultimately, training and tuning represent not merely different methods but divergent relationships with the body—one of control versus dialogue, objectification versus embodiment. Recognising and integrating these dimensions enriches the landscape of movement practice, offering pathways to performance that honour the body's intelligence and support holistic wellbeing. This subchapter invites readers to reconsider their own movement practices through the lens of tuning, opening to a deeper, more responsive engagement with the body that transcends mere mechanics and touches the essence of embodied life.

Play, Flow, and the Forgotten Joy of Movement

The impulse to move spontaneously, playfully, and joyfully is often dismissed in adulthood as trivial or unproductive—a vestige of childhood that must be outgrown in favour of discipline, efficiency, and goal-directed effort. Yet this cultural relegation overlooks a fundamental truth: playful movement is not mere frivolity, but a foundational aspect of human wellbeing and development. The joyous, unstructured engagement with the body that defines play nurtures creativity, emotional regulation, and social connection. Complementing this is Mihaly Csikszentmihalyi's seminal concept of *flow*, a state of optimal experience characterised by absorption, challenge, and intrinsic reward. Together, the psychology of play and the neuroscience of flow reveal that joyful, spontaneous movement is central not only to childhood development but to lifelong psychological health and embodied flourishing.

Play, as developmental psychology establishes, is the crucible in which motor skills, emotional resilience, and social competence are forged. From the uncoordinated tumble of infants to the complex games of older children, play offers a space for experimentation, risk-taking, and mastery without the pressure of external evaluation. Movement play engages the whole organism, integrating sensorimotor systems with affective and cognitive processes. This holistic engagement fosters neural plasticity, enhances interoceptive awareness, and builds the capacity for adaptive emotional responses. Far from being a mere precursor to "serious" activity, play lays the groundwork for adaptive movement patterns and emotional regulation that support adult wellbeing.

Csikszentmihalyi's flow theory elucidates why certain movement experiences captivate and sustain us, transcending mundane exercise to become deeply rewarding. Flow occurs when a person is fully immersed in an activity that balances challenge with skill, generating a sense of effortless control, altered time perception, and loss of self-consciousness. Physical activities such as dancing, climbing, or surfing commonly induce flow, as do more quotidian embodied engagements when approached with presence. Flow's neurological correlates—heightened connectivity between attention, motor, and reward systems—suggest that it optimises brain function and promotes positive affect. The experience of flow through movement is thus a powerful antidote to disconnection and psychological distress.

The adult abandonment of play and flow is culturally shaped by values privileging productivity, control, and external achievement. This shift contributes to a widespread disembodiment marked by sedentary lifestyles and an impoverished relationship with movement. Yet reclaiming play and flow is both possible and essential. Emerging movements in somatic education, improvisational dance, and adventure sports emphasise the restoration of spontaneous, joyful movement as a pathway to health. For instance, practitioners of Contact Improvisation explore movement as a playful, relational art, highlighting how shared physical play fosters emotional attunement and creativity. Similarly, parkour enthusiasts re-engage with their environments through playful exploration, exemplifying how flow states arise from dynamic, adaptive movement.

Playful movement and flow are not merely recreational; they are foundational to embodied intelligence and psychological integration. By engaging the body in joyful exploration, we cultivate a somatic wisdom that informs emotional regulation and cognitive flexibility. This somatic attunement enriches self-awareness and fosters resilience in the face of stress. Moreover, play and flow disrupt habitual, rigid movement patterns and mental schemas, enabling renewal and growth. They invite a reimagining of exercise and physical activity as creative, expressive practices that nourish the whole person.

Critically, the revalorisation of play and flow challenges the commodification of fitness and the reduction of movement to mechanistic training. Instead of movement as obligation or chore, it foregrounds movement as a source of intrinsic joy and meaning. This shift has implications for mental health, education, and community life, suggesting that spaces and cultures supporting playful, flow-inducing movement can counteract the alienation and fragmentation characteristic of modern living.

Ethically, embracing play and flow requires attending to accessibility and inclusivity. Not all bodies and minds have equal opportunity for spontaneous movement due to disability, social marginalisation, or trauma. Designing environments and practices that invite diverse forms of play and flow is therefore crucial. This commitment honours the universal human right to embodied joy and aliveness, transcending limitations imposed by social or physical constraints.

In practical terms, cultivating play and flow involves re-engaging with the body's natural rhythms and curiosity. Simple acts—dancing alone, exploring new movement patterns, or engaging in improvisational games—can ignite the conditions for flow and the vitality of play. These practices cultivate presence, soften self-judgment, and reconnect individuals to the pleasure and power of their bodies.

Ultimately, play and flow reclaim movement's rightful place as a cornerstone of psychological health and embodied wisdom. Far from incidental or indulgent, they constitute fundamental modes of being that enrich life's texture and resilience. By revisiting these dimensions, this chapter invites readers to rediscover the forgotten joy of movement—a joy that sustains creativity, connection, and the profound aliveness at the heart of the human experience.

Reclaiming Movement from Capitalism

Movement, in its most primal and human form, is a birthright—an innate capacity for expression, connection, and survival. Yet, under the pervasive influence of capitalist economies and consumer culture, this fundamental human experience has been transformed into a commodity, packaged, marketed, and sold as a lifestyle or product to be purchased. The commodification of fitness distorts movement's essence, shifting its meaning from embodied joy and health to a transaction defined by external standards, status, and profit. This subchapter undertakes a critical examination of how capitalist logics have shaped contemporary fitness culture and offers a compelling reframing: movement as an irreducible human right, essential to psychological and social wellbeing, and inherently resistant to commodification.

The fitness industry today is a multi-billion-dollar enterprise, saturating media, retail, and digital platforms with promises of transformation through consumption—whether of gym memberships, branded apparel, supplements, or regimented programmes. This commercial apparatus relies on perpetuating insecurities about body image, health, and worth, creating a cycle of demand that privileges appearance and performance as markers of success. Movement is instrumentalised, reduced to a means for producing marketable bodies rather than experienced as a source of vitality and autonomy. This commodification not only alienates individuals from the pleasure of movement but also exacerbates inequities, as access to "fitness" becomes increasingly stratified by socioeconomic status.

Critical analysis reveals that this phenomenon is not incidental but structurally embedded within capitalist modes of production and consumption. The industry thrives on creating desires rather than meeting needs, turning movement into a spectacle and lifestyle brand that demands ongoing investment and adherence. Fitness becomes performative, a mode of self-branding and social distinction rather than a spontaneous or self-directed activity. The resultant culture valorises discipline, control, and consumption, often at the expense of holistic wellbeing and authentic embodiment. In this context, the body risks becoming a project of optimisation and display, disconnected from its intrinsic rhythms and needs.

Contrasting sharply with this commercialised paradigm are diverse cultural and historical practices that honour movement as communal, ritualistic, and regenerative. Indigenous dances, communal celebrations, and traditional physical practices embody movement as collective expression, spiritual communion, and social cohesion—activities inseparable from identity and belonging. These forms resist commodification by foregrounding relationality, meaning, and accessibility. They remind us that movement's deepest value lies not in spectacle or marketability but in its capacity to connect individuals to themselves, each other, and the world.

The reclamation of movement from capitalism requires both personal and political engagement. On an individual level, it involves cultivating awareness of the ways in which consumer culture shapes attitudes toward the body and movement, and intentionally resisting reductionist narratives. Practices such as free-form dance, unstructured play, and somatic exploration offer pathways to rediscover movement as intrinsic expression rather than obligation or performance. These modalities emphasise *presence* and *joy*, dismantling the dichotomy between exercise as work and movement as pleasure.

Politically, reclaiming movement calls for challenging systemic barriers that limit access to safe, welcoming spaces for embodied activity. Socioeconomic disparities, ableism, and cultural exclusions restrict who can participate in fitness culture and how. Movements for body positivity, inclusive recreation, and community-based physical activity contest the monopolisation of movement by capitalist and normative frameworks. They advocate for democratizing movement as a public good and cultural commons, affirming its role in social justice and health equity.

Real-world examples of this reclamation abound. Community dance projects that invite participants of all ages and abilities celebrate movement as collective joy rather than performance. Urban skateboarding cultures repurpose public spaces for creative expression and social connection outside commercial or institutional control. Grassroots initiatives offering free or low-cost movement classes in underserved neighbourhoods exemplify efforts to decouple movement from commodification and privilege. These practices enact the reframing of movement as accessible, relational, and emancipatory.

Reclaiming movement also demands a critical interrogation of technology's role. While digital platforms and wearable devices offer new opportunities for engagement and data-driven self-awareness, they can also reinforce commodification by fostering surveillance, comparison, and algorithm-driven consumption. Navigating these tensions requires mindful integration of technology that supports embodied presence rather than performance anxiety or consumerist impulse.

Ethically, this reclamation underscores the importance of honouring bodily autonomy, diversity, and dignity. Movement as birthright entails recognizing varied ways of moving and being in the world, rejecting one-size-fits-all ideals imposed by commercial fitness. It demands spaces that are safe, inclusive, and affirming of difference—whether in age, ability, culture, or identity.

In reframing movement away from capitalist commodification and toward embodied birthright, this chapter invites readers to rediscover the profound and liberatory dimensions of movement. It calls for reclaiming movement as an act of self-care, creative expression, and social belonging—fundamental to health and happiness beyond market metrics. Such reclamation is not a nostalgic return but a visionary engagement with movement's potential to restore wholeness, agency, and connection in a world often fractured by commodification and alienation.

Chapter 6
Motion Sickness—When Movement Triggers Malaise

Exercise is often praised as one of the most reliable foundations of health, celebrated for its capacity to strengthen the body, elevate mood, and fend off illness. The story is so familiar it risks becoming dogma. Yet beneath this narrative lies a disquieting paradox: for some, movement does not soothe but unsettles. Instead of dissolving stress, it sharpens it. Rather than lifting spirits, it can stir unease, dysregulation, even echoes of old trauma. This chapter turns its attention to that tension—the phenomenon of exercise-induced malaise—where activity intended to restore vitality instead unsettles the very systems it is meant to support. In drawing apart these contradictions, we begin to see movement not as a monolithic cure but as a practice woven with complexity.

Episodes of heightened anxiety or restlessness after exercise reveal a different physiological truth: unresolved trauma, adrenal overdrive, or a sensitised nervous system may cause activity to inflame, not soothe. A brisk run or high-intensity session, for one person liberating, may for another bring on panic, exhaustion, or fragmentation. This is not weakness but physiology at work. Such patterns unsettle the easy refrain that "exercise helps everyone" and press us towards trauma-informed, personalised approaches. Research from trauma studies and psychophysiology underscores the point: the body remembers. Past wounds, lodged beneath awareness, can be jolted awake by certain kinds of exertion. To pretend otherwise is to strip exercise of its subtlety.

Layered upon this is the perfectionism trap so deeply embedded in contemporary fitness culture. The endless chase for idealised physiques, faultless performance, and rigid discipline often disguises an inner hunger for control, or a way of outrunning disquiet. What presents as dedication may, in truth, be compulsion. For many, exercise becomes less a practice of care than an escape from pain—a coping mechanism that, ironically, deepens fatigue, alienation, or distorted self-image. The very culture that prizes endurance and grit risks cementing a cycle where movement both consoles and confines. To interrogate this dynamic is to expose the unspoken costs of our cultural obsession with mastery over the body.

Equally insidious is the culture of toxic positivity that saturates many training environments. Phrases like "no pain, no gain" or "push through" masquerade as motivation, yet they often silence vulnerability and invalidate authentic bodily feedback. Discomfort is conflated with growth, and pain is lauded as proof of progress. Lost in this rhetoric is the truth that not all strain is transformative. A more humane framework draws instead on emotional intelligence: listening to sensation, honouring limits, pacing with compassion. Such alternatives invite a return to nuance—acknowledging that resilience is not brute endurance but the capacity to remain present with what the body is actually saying.

Against this backdrop, the value of stillness and restorative practices deserves emphasis. Movement does not always heal; sometimes the deepest medicine is found in quiet. Breathwork, restorative yoga, Tension & Trauma Releasing Exercises—these slower, gentler approaches foster regulation and integration, giving the nervous system a chance to reset. They remind us that embodied wellbeing is not a ladder of exertion to be climbed endlessly upward, but a rhythm between doing and undoing, arousal and release.

What emerges, then, is a more textured understanding of movement's paradoxes. This chapter does not discard the immense value of exercise but insists on recognising its double edge: healing and harm, vitality and disruption, play out differently across bodies and histories. It calls for humility, for willingness to move past binaries of good and bad, and to meet exercise with discernment.

For practitioners, educators, or anyone seeking to inhabit their body with integrity, the invitation is clear: cultivate practices that honour variation, welcome vulnerability, and prioritise care over performance. Such a shift demands that we dismantle the cultural myths of toughness and uniformity, making space instead for trauma-informed, emotionally intelligent movement cultures. Rest, after all, is not surrender. Attunement is not weakness. Both may be acts of radical strength.

In reclaiming these truths, we loosen the grip of fitness dogma and restore exercise to what it might be at its best: not an imposed regimen but a responsive, deeply human practice—capable of wounding, yes, but also of healing when approached with attentiveness, honesty, and respect.

Exercise-Induced Anxiety and Dysregulation

Exercise is widely championed as a powerful tool for managing anxiety and enhancing mental health. The conventional wisdom is straightforward: physical activity stimulates endorphin release, regulates stress hormones, and promotes neuroplasticity, all contributing to improved mood and emotional resilience. However, this narrative, while valid for many, masks a paradoxical reality for a significant subset of individuals who experience heightened anxiety and physiological dysregulation following exercise. Understanding this phenomenon requires an exploration of the complex interplay between unresolved trauma, adrenal function, and the nervous system's response to bodily activation—an intersection where movement can inadvertently trigger distress rather than relief.

At the core of exercise-induced anxiety lies the body's stress response, governed primarily by the autonomic nervous system (ANS). Exercise, particularly of moderate to high intensity, activates the sympathetic branch of the ANS, increasing heart rate, blood pressure, and cortisol secretion. For most, this physiological arousal is transient and balanced by parasympathetic recovery, resulting in homeostasis and enhanced wellbeing. Yet, for individuals with chronic stress or trauma histories, this balance is disrupted. Their nervous systems may already be sensitised or dysregulated, primed for hypervigilance and exaggerated threat perception. In such cases, exercise-induced sympathetic activation can overload these fragile systems, precipitating heightened anxiety, panic attacks, or prolonged dysregulation.

Clinical observations and emerging research highlight this dynamic. Studies reveal that trauma survivors—especially those with post-traumatic stress disorder (PTSD)—often report increased anxiety, racing heartbeats, or dissociative episodes post-exercise. The physiological cues of exertion mimic those of danger, triggering conditioned fear responses. This somatic flashback phenomenon underscores how unresolved trauma is embodied, embedded in neurophysiological patterns that are reactivated by bodily arousal. Thus, while exercise theoretically should soothe stress, it paradoxically serves as a somatic trigger, intensifying anxiety symptoms.

Another critical factor is adrenal health and its role in regulating the stress hormone cascade. Chronic stress or overtraining can lead to adrenal fatigue or dysregulation, marked by impaired cortisol rhythms and blunted stress responses. Paradoxically, this state can manifest as both exhaustion and heightened anxiety. The body's diminished capacity to buffer stress exacerbates post-exercise malaise, resulting in persistent nervous system arousal and impaired recovery. For these individuals, conventional exercise prescriptions may be counterproductive, necessitating carefully calibrated approaches that prioritise nervous system regulation over intensity or volume.

This nuanced understanding challenges the simplistic notion that more exercise unequivocally equates to better mental health. It calls for a trauma-informed, individualised framework that recognises the diversity of responses to physical activity. Such a framework integrates awareness of personal history, neurophysiological patterns, and current capacity, guiding practitioners and individuals toward movement modalities and intensities that support regulation rather than dysregulation.

Practically, this approach entails incorporating pacing, grounding techniques, and somatic awareness into exercise routines. Mindful movement practices—such as yoga, tai chi, or restorative stretching—can facilitate gentle activation coupled with parasympathetic engagement, fostering neurophysiological balance. Breath regulation and interoceptive attention empower individuals to monitor and respond to their internal states, preventing overwhelm. In therapeutic contexts, somatic experiencing and sensorimotor psychotherapy employ movement and touch to renegotiate trauma imprints safely, highlighting the centrality of embodied regulation.

The broader fitness culture often overlooks or minimises these complexities, promoting uniform exercise models and neglecting the embodied narratives of those for whom movement triggers distress. This oversight perpetuates stigma and discouragement, as individuals internalise difficulties as personal failure rather than manifestations of physiological and psychological processes. Shifting cultural narratives to normalise diverse responses to exercise is essential for inclusive and compassionate health promotion.

Research is beginning to illuminate biomarkers and predictive indicators for exercise-induced dysregulation, opening avenues for tailored interventions. Heart rate variability monitoring, cortisol assays, and psychophysiological assessments offer objective data to personalise exercise prescriptions. However, technology must be paired with attuned clinical and personal insight to avoid reductive or mechanistic interpretations.

Ethically, recognising exercise-induced anxiety demands humility and responsiveness from practitioners, trainers, and healthcare providers. It challenges one-size-fits-all prescriptions and emphasises client autonomy, safety, and collaboration. Trauma-informed movement education and coaching cultivate environments where vulnerability is honoured and pacing is respected, enabling gradual reclamation of embodied wellbeing.

In summary, exercise-induced anxiety and dysregulation reveal the intricate, sometimes paradoxical relationship between movement and mental health. They underscore the imperative to move beyond reductive, universalistic models toward frameworks that integrate trauma science, neurophysiology, and embodied practice. Embracing this complexity enriches our understanding and cultivates pathways to movement that heal rather than harm—affirming the body's wisdom and resilience amid challenge.

The Perfectionism Trap

Compulsive fitness culture, with its relentless pursuit of ideal bodies and peak performance, often masks a deeper psychological phenomenon: emotional avoidance cloaked in discipline and perfectionism. At first glance, rigorous exercise routines and strict dietary regimens may seem like healthy commitments to self-care, but beneath the surface, they can function as strategies to evade uncomfortable feelings, unresolved trauma, or relational difficulties. This dynamic, commonly referred to as the *perfectionism trap*, not only distorts the relationship with the body but also exacerbates conditions such as body dysmorphia and social disconnection. To understand this trap is to unravel how cultural ideals, psychological defence mechanisms, and embodied experience intersect within contemporary fitness practices.

Perfectionism in fitness culture manifests as a compulsive striving for flawlessness—not only in physical form but also in routines, performance metrics, and lifestyle choices. This drive often derives from internalised messages equating worth with achievement and control, reflecting broader sociocultural norms that valorise discipline and productivity. While goal orientation and commitment are valuable, perfectionism introduces rigidity and self-criticism that undermine genuine wellbeing. The body, once a source of pleasure and vitality, becomes a battleground where failure to meet unrealistic standards triggers shame, anxiety, and a vicious cycle of overexertion.

Psychologically, compulsive fitness behaviours serve as coping mechanisms for difficult emotional states. Rather than directly engaging with feelings such as grief, loneliness, or fear, individuals may channel energy into regimented exercise and dietary control as means of distraction or self-soothing. This form of emotional avoidance, while temporarily effective, ultimately inhibits authentic emotional processing and self-integration. The body's needs and signals are overridden by cognitive scripts prioritising achievement and appearance, resulting in disconnection from embodied wisdom and increased vulnerability to distress.

Body dysmorphia—a distorted perception of one's body—often intensifies within this perfectionism framework. Individuals become fixated on perceived flaws, no matter how minor or unfounded, and interpret their bodies through a lens of defectiveness. This preoccupation fuels compulsive behaviours aimed at 'fixing' the body, reinforcing negative self-evaluation and perpetuating the cycle.

The rise of social media and digitally mediated fitness culture amplifies these dynamics, exposing individuals to curated images and narratives that elevate unattainable ideals and foster comparison. The relentless exposure to such content exacerbates body dissatisfaction and heightens perfectionistic tendencies.

Relational detachment is another significant consequence of the perfectionism trap. The obsessive focus on self-regulation and control can undermine interpersonal connection, as emotional vulnerability is feared or repressed. Fitness routines may become isolating rituals, prioritising solitary exertion over social engagement. This withdrawal reinforces loneliness and diminishes the support networks essential for holistic health. Paradoxically, the very practices intended to enhance wellbeing can entrench patterns of disconnection and emotional numbness.

Contemporary fitness culture's glorification of "no pain, no gain" and "push through" mantras exemplifies toxic perfectionism, valorising suffering as proof of commitment and dismissing bodily or emotional limits. Such narratives delegitimise pain, fatigue, or ambivalence, pressuring individuals to ignore warning signs and perpetuate unsustainable behaviours. This toxic positivity silences authentic experience and perpetuates harm, creating environments where shame and exhaustion thrive behind façades of discipline.

Countering the perfectionism trap requires embracing a more compassionate, embodied approach to movement and self-care. Somatic therapies, mindful movement practices, and trauma-informed coaching foster attunement to bodily signals and emotional states, disrupting compulsive cycles. These modalities encourage curiosity, acceptance, and flexibility—qualities antithetical to perfectionism but foundational for integration and healing. By reorienting movement toward dialogue rather than domination, individuals can reclaim agency and foster wholeness.

Critical reflection also entails interrogating cultural narratives that valorise perfectionism and commodify fitness ideals. Questioning who benefits from perpetuating unrealistic standards and exploring alternative models of health and embodiment opens space for more inclusive, humane approaches. Community-based movement initiatives, body-positive campaigns, and inclusive fitness environments exemplify efforts to dismantle perfectionism's grip and cultivate diverse expressions of embodied wellbeing.

Ethically, acknowledging the harms of compulsive fitness culture demands responsiveness from practitioners, educators, and industry leaders. Creating spaces that prioritise psychological safety, encourage vulnerability, and resist commodification is essential for fostering authentic connection and healing. This includes recognising the intersectional factors—such as gender, race, and socioeconomic status—that shape experiences of body image and perfectionism, ensuring equity in access and representation.

Ultimately, the perfectionism trap reveals how movement practices can obscure rather than reveal the self when co-opted by fear and avoidance. Understanding this dynamic invites a profound reconsideration of fitness culture, urging a shift from external validation toward internal attunement. It challenges individuals and societies to cultivate movement not as punishment or performance but as an expressive, nurturing, and integrative practice—one that honours imperfection as intrinsic to human embodiment and flourishing.

Toxic Positivity in Fitness Spaces

The prevailing culture of fitness often elevates motivational slogans to dogma—catchphrases like "no pain, no gain" or "push through the burn" are ubiquitous, repeated ad nauseam in gyms, social media feeds, and coaching sessions. These affirmations, while ostensibly designed to inspire, frequently function as vehicles of *toxic positivity*: a relentless insistence on maintaining a cheerful, can-do attitude that dismisses, minimises, or invalidates genuine emotional experience. This phenomenon presents significant challenges for those engaging in movement as a path to wellbeing, as it not only obscures the complexities of embodied life but also perpetuates harm by silencing vulnerability, discouraging authentic self-awareness, and fostering unrealistic expectations. To grapple with toxic positivity in fitness spaces is to confront how cultural scripts around motivation intersect with power, emotion, and embodiment—and to envision alternatives grounded in emotional intelligence and compassionate coaching.

Toxic positivity, in its essence, denies the full spectrum of human experience by privileging optimism and performance over authenticity and self-compassion. Within fitness contexts, this often translates into an environment where discomfort, fatigue, doubt, or emotional struggle are perceived as weakness or failure. The injunction to "just keep going" or "embrace the pain" becomes a form of emotional censorship, pressuring individuals to mask distress and conform to an idealised narrative of relentless perseverance. This dynamic not only invalidates the embodied signals that may indicate the need for rest or recalibration but also cultivates shame around natural variations in energy, motivation, and mood.

Such rhetoric carries particularly pernicious effects when directed toward those with histories of trauma, chronic illness, or mental health challenges. For these individuals, the body's signals are often complex and fraught, and the demand to maintain positivity or endure discomfort without question can exacerbate dysregulation, anxiety, or injury. Clinical practitioners and somatic therapists increasingly recognise that movement practices divorced from emotional attunement risk re-traumatisation or alienation. The insistence on "powering through" neglects the vital role of pacing, attunement, and listening in sustainable embodied wellbeing.

The critique of toxic positivity also intersects with broader cultural patterns that valorise productivity, individual responsibility, and control. Fitness spaces, as microcosms of neoliberal ideals, often frame effort and success as entirely contingent on willpower and attitude. This framing obscures social determinants of health, systemic inequities, and the multifaceted nature of wellbeing. By reducing complex embodied experiences to simplistic narratives of grit, toxic positivity perpetuates exclusion and marginalisation. Those who do not conform to the idealised fitness persona—due to disability, age, body size, or neurodiversity—may find themselves further alienated or pathologised.

Reimagining fitness culture requires cultivating emotionally intelligent coaching and community environments that honour vulnerability, nuance, and embodied wisdom. Emotionally intelligent coaching recognises that motivation is not a static trait but a dynamic interplay of cognitive, affective, and somatic factors. It invites clients to engage with their internal experiences openly, to honour discomfort as information, and to co-create movement practices that balance challenge with care. Such approaches draw on psychological theories of self-compassion, interoception, and trauma-informed care, integrating them into embodied practice.

Real-world applications of emotionally intelligent coaching demonstrate its transformative potential. For example, in trauma-sensitive yoga programs, instructors explicitly acknowledge the validity of participants' emotional states and encourage pacing and choice, dismantling the "push through" imperative. Similarly, strength coaches working with athletes recovering from injury increasingly incorporate psychological readiness and embodied feedback into training plans, fostering resilience without coercion. These models shift the locus of control from external achievement to internal attunement, enhancing both performance and wellbeing.

The language used in fitness spaces also plays a critical role in perpetuating or countering toxic positivity. Replacing combative metaphors ("battle," "fight," "warrior") with language that emphasises collaboration, curiosity, and self-kindness can create a more inclusive and sustainable culture. Encouraging expressions of frustration, doubt, or fatigue as normal aspects of embodied life helps dismantle stigma and builds psychological safety.

Technology and social media, double-edged tools in contemporary fitness culture, contribute both to the spread of toxic positivity and to its contestation. Online communities can amplify idealised portrayals of fitness success, fostering comparison and perfectionism. Yet they also provide platforms for vulnerability, peer support, and alternative narratives that challenge mainstream fitness ideologies. Harnessing these digital spaces to promote emotionally intelligent discourse and diverse embodiments is a crucial frontier.

Ethically, addressing toxic positivity entails acknowledging the power dynamics embedded in fitness spaces and advocating for equity and inclusion. Recognising whose voices are amplified or silenced, whose bodies are celebrated or marginalised, and how cultural narratives intersect with identity factors such as gender, race, and class is essential for fostering truly supportive environments.

In sum, toxic positivity in fitness spaces is a pervasive but surmountable barrier to authentic embodied wellbeing. By interrogating its cultural roots and psychological impacts, and by cultivating emotionally intelligent, compassionate approaches to movement, we can transform fitness from a site of pressure and denial into a space of genuine connection, healing, and flourishing. This shift honours the complexity of human experience and restores movement's capacity to nourish body, mind, and spirit in profound and sustainable ways.

When Stillness is Healing

The dominant discourse surrounding movement and wellbeing often privileges activity, exertion, and progress—encouraging us to see physical motion as inherently beneficial and stillness as, at best, passive or, at worst, lazy. Yet this prevailing narrative obscures a vital truth: *not all movement is healing*, and sometimes the most transformative interventions come from intentional rest, breath, and slow, mindful practices. In a culture that equates motion with vitality and stagnation with failure, reclaiming the power of stillness as a pathway to integration and recovery demands a profound recalibration of our relationship to the body and mind.

The therapeutic potential of stillness emerges most clearly when examined through the lens of nervous system regulation. Our autonomic nervous system (ANS) oscillates between states of arousal and relaxation, sympathetic activation and parasympathetic rest. While movement, especially vigorous exercise, can catalyse sympathetic engagement necessary for survival and resilience, healing from trauma, chronic stress, or dysregulation often requires the restorative embrace of parasympathetic activation. Intentional stillness—embodied in slow breath, gentle stretching, or supported postures—facilitates this shift, allowing the nervous system to downregulate, process stored tension, and foster neurochemical balance.

Restorative yoga exemplifies how slow, mindful practices can nurture this healing process. Unlike more intense forms of yoga that challenge strength and flexibility, restorative yoga employs prolonged holds supported by props to cultivate deep muscular and nervous system relaxation. Clinical studies confirm its efficacy in reducing anxiety, improving sleep, and modulating stress hormones, demonstrating that stillness is far from inert; it is an active engagement with embodied presence. This practice invites participants to cultivate radical acceptance and to meet their bodies with gentleness—a potent antidote to the relentless "push harder" ethos pervading much of fitness culture.

Similarly, Tension & Trauma Releasing Exercises (TRE) illustrate the profound somatic effects of intentional stillness coupled with subtle movement. Developed by trauma specialist David Berceli, TRE activates the body's natural tremor mechanism, allowing involuntary shaking that facilitates the release of deep muscular tension and trauma-related holding patterns. This approach is neither passive nor forceful but arises from the body's innate wisdom, demonstrating how calibrated stillness intertwined with spontaneous movement can restore resilience. TRE highlights the importance of listening to the body's spontaneous impulses rather than imposing externally dictated movement regimes.

Breathwork, another cornerstone of stillness-based healing, engages the autonomic nervous system through deliberate modulation of respiration patterns. Slow, diaphragmatic breathing stimulates the vagus nerve, enhances heart rate variability, and promotes emotional regulation. Practices such as pranayama, coherent breathing, or the Wim Hof Method differ in technique but share the capacity to transform physiological and psychological states through conscious stillness. By centring attention on breath, individuals cultivate *interoception*—a heightened awareness of internal bodily sensations—that deepens self-connection and equips them to navigate stress with greater resilience.

Importantly, embracing stillness as healing challenges dominant cultural valuations of productivity and constant activation. Our society often pathologises rest as weakness or idleness, marginalising those who require slower, more nuanced rhythms for health. This bias is particularly pronounced in the context of trauma recovery or chronic illness, where overexertion can exacerbate symptoms and prolong suffering. Recognising the legitimacy of stillness as an essential, active component of healing calls for dismantling stigmas and expanding definitions of health to encompass diverse embodied experiences.

Real-world applications of stillness-based healing are increasingly evident across clinical, therapeutic, and community settings. Trauma-informed yoga programmes in veterans' hospitals, mindfulness-based stress reduction courses in cancer care, and somatic therapies for survivors of abuse all centre stillness and gentle movement as foundational modalities. These interventions demonstrate measurable benefits in reducing PTSD symptoms, chronic pain, and depression, underscoring the necessity of integrating stillness alongside more active practices in holistic health models.

Stillness also functions as a profound psychological counterbalance to the overstimulation of modern life. In a world saturated with digital noise, rapid pace, and constant demands, cultivating embodied stillness provides a sanctuary for reflection, emotional processing, and somatic integration. This capacity is not synonymous with passivity but represents a dynamic state of receptivity, groundedness, and openness to experience. It equips individuals to move through life with greater clarity, intention, and adaptive flexibility.

Ethically, privileging stillness as healing entails advocating for accessible spaces and practices that honour diverse needs and rhythms. This includes addressing barriers to rest, such as socioeconomic constraints, caregiving responsibilities, or cultural imperatives that valorise busyness. Creating environments—whether in healthcare, workplaces, or communities—that respect and facilitate restorative practices is essential for fostering equitable wellbeing.

Furthermore, stillness invites a philosophical re-examination of what it means to *move well.* It challenges reductionist views that equate movement solely with physical exertion or aesthetic performance, expanding the definition to encompass mindful presence, somatic attunement, and relational engagement with the self. This reorientation aligns with embodied cognition research demonstrating that cognition and affect emerge from dynamic interactions between body and environment, in which stillness plays a vital integrative role.

In sum, recognising when stillness is healing enriches our understanding of movement's full spectrum and challenges cultural biases privileging action over rest. Intentional stillness—through restorative yoga, breathwork, TRE, and related modalities—offers powerful pathways for nervous system regulation, trauma recovery, and emotional resilience. This chapter encourages readers to embrace stillness not as an absence of movement but as a deeply active, transformative practice central to embodied wellbeing and wholeness.

Chapter 7
Collective Bodies, Collective Moods

Human beings are, at their core, creatures of relation—our emotions rarely confined to private interiors but constantly entangled with the gestures, rhythms, and presences of others. Place us in a crowd and the lines between self and collective begin to soften: not only do our bodies share space, but our moods, pulses, and energies slip into alignment. This chapter traces that phenomenon of emotional entrainment—the way synchronised movement within groups, whether at a protest march, a music festival, or a regimented drill, recalibrates neural rhythms and fuses individuals into something larger than themselves. What emerges in such moments is not merely a sum of discrete feelings, but a fabric of collective affect where movement becomes a powerful conductor of emotion and cohesion.

At the heart of this lies our nervous system's inherent tendency toward resonance. The discovery of mirror neurons in the 1990s offered a glimpse of the mechanics: when we observe the gestures or postures of others, our brains light up as though performing them ourselves. This is not a trivial reflex. It is one of the most basic architectures of empathy, communication, and belonging. Hence why moving together—whether in the tactical coordination of a football team, the ritual gestures of a congregation, or the chant-driven march of demonstrators—creates a solidarity that words alone cannot summon.

Movement as a language of belonging is hardly new. Across time and culture, carefully choreographed dances, repetitive ritual gestures, and synchronised sporting acts have marked the boundaries of community and reaffirmed values held in common. A dance troupe's precision, a monastery's bowing, a team's rehearsed play: each performs more than action, each embodies trust, interdependence, or devotion. Here, meaning does not sit in abstract symbols but in embodied cognition—knowledge lodged in muscle, rhythm, and breath, in the lived sensation of moving as one.

Yet to imagine collective movement solely as harmony is to miss half its power. Bodies in synchrony can resist as forcefully as they can unite. History is full of moments when those denied voice or visibility turned to movement as defiance. Think of the civil rights marches, where walking itself became a public proclamation of dignity and justice. Or Capoeira in Brazil, part dance, part combat, part ritual—a disguised rebellion against colonial power, preserving culture under the guise of play. In such instances, bodies do not simply express dissent; they enact it, creating a choreography of resistance written into the flesh of history.

Nor is this power confined to politics. Communal movement has long carried within it the possibility of collective healing. Indigenous drumming circles, African grief rituals, modern therapeutic dance practices—all deploy rhythm and motion to metabolise pain and knit fractured bonds. Within these circles, people breathe, sway, drum, or weep together, and in doing so, regulate one another's nervous systems. Neuroscience lends weight to what practitioners already knew: rhythmic motion can boost oxytocin, regulate vagal tone, and restore emotional equilibrium. Healing here is not metaphor but physiology—the body re-learning safety through the presence of other bodies.

Contemporary life offers its own secular rituals. Vast crowds at concerts, stadiums, or festivals move in unison—sometimes choreographed, sometimes spontaneous—and through that shared movement experience emotions that are magnified, contagious, and unforgettable. Joy, grief, protest, solidarity: each finds amplification in the synchrony of many bodies. These experiences often reshape identity itself, fusing the personal with the communal, revealing how our social fabric is stitched not only with words but with steps, beats, and gestures.

Yet, as with all potent forces, there is a shadow side. The same entrainment that binds can also unleash panic, rage, or despair, as seen in stampedes or violent riots. Here the synchrony of bodies does not console but destabilises. Which direction collective movement takes—toward cohesion or chaos—depends heavily on context, leadership, and intention. The ethical stakes are not trivial.

This chapter therefore pulls from neuroscience, anthropology, psychology, and political thought to chart a fuller picture of collective embodiment. It suggests that emotions and cognition cannot be understood as isolated processes but are constantly sculpted in relation with others. To move together is to think and feel together, sometimes in ways we cannot quite name.

By its conclusion, the reader will have seen how collective bodies—whether swaying in ritual, marching in protest, or dancing in ecstasy—compose living tapestries of shared memory and mood. The challenge, and the invitation, is to move with greater awareness: to cultivate forms of collective synchrony that connect, restore, and liberate rather than fragment. In a fractured age, this may be one of the most radical gestures we have.

Contagious Motion, Contagious Emotion

The phenomenon of emotional contagion—the seamless, often unconscious transmission of feelings from one individual to another—is as old as human society itself. When entwined with synchronized physical movement, this process becomes a powerful force that shapes collective mood, identity, and action. The concept of *emotional entrainment* captures this dynamic interplay, describing how rhythmic coordination in groups—whether during protests, concerts, or military drills—not only aligns bodies but also aligns affective states, forging a shared emotional landscape that transcends individual experience. Understanding emotional entrainment invites us to reconsider how movement functions as a foundational medium of social cohesion, collective identity, and communal resilience.

At the neurological level, emotional entrainment is rooted in the brain's inherent capacity for synchronization. Mirror neuron systems, discovered in the late 20th century, reveal that observing or engaging in movement activates neural circuits that facilitate empathy and mimicry. This neural mirroring enables individuals to resonate with others' emotions through shared motion, effectively creating a neural feedback loop that amplifies group affect. For instance, studies employing electroencephalography (EEG) have demonstrated that participants engaged in coordinated activities exhibit synchronized brainwave patterns, particularly in areas associated with social cognition and emotional regulation. These findings underscore the embodied nature of social connection: *we literally feel each other's emotions through movement.*

Real-world examples vividly illustrate emotional entrainment's potency. Consider the collective effervescence observed at large-scale protests. Participants moving in unison—marching, chanting, raising fists—experience a heightened sense of solidarity and shared purpose. This embodied unity can catalyse emotional states ranging from empowered joy to righteous anger, fueling collective action. Similarly, at music festivals or religious ceremonies, rhythmic dancing and chanting synchronize participants' movements and heart rates, fostering feelings of belonging and transcendence. Military drills, with their precise, regimented coordination, generate a distinct collective mood of discipline and readiness, embedding a shared identity among soldiers.

Yet emotional entrainment is not confined to large crowds; it operates in smaller, everyday interactions. Conversational gestures, postural mimicry, and synchronized walking between friends or colleagues subtly influence mood and rapport. This micro-level entrainment lays the groundwork for broader social harmonies or tensions, demonstrating how movement and emotion are continuously co-constructed within interpersonal spaces. The embodied feedback loop—where emotion drives movement, which in turn shapes emotion—underscores the bidirectional, dynamic nature of human connection.

The power of emotional entrainment extends beyond social bonding to influence decision-making and group dynamics. Neuroscientific research suggests that synchronized movement enhances trust, cooperation, and pro-social behaviour, which are critical for collective problem-solving and resilience. For example, experimental paradigms involving synchronized finger tapping or rowing have shown increased willingness among participants to share resources or coordinate efforts. These findings have profound implications for organisational leadership, therapeutic interventions, and community building, highlighting how fostering embodied synchrony can cultivate more cohesive and effective groups.

However, emotional entrainment is a double-edged sword. While it can promote solidarity and healing, it also has the capacity to escalate collective fear, aggression, or panic. Historical events such as riots or mass hysteria exemplify how synchronized emotional states, when unregulated, can lead to destructive outcomes. This ambivalence calls for ethical reflection on how entrainment is facilitated, highlighting the importance of context, intention, and leadership in guiding collective affect. Understanding the mechanisms and boundaries of emotional contagion equips communities to harness its benefits while mitigating risks.

Philosophically, emotional entrainment challenges entrenched dualisms separating mind and body, individual and collective. It reveals that cognition and affect are fundamentally relational and embodied, shaped through dynamic interactions among moving bodies. This perspective aligns with contemporary theories of embodied cognition and enactivism, which argue that knowledge and emotion arise from embodied engagement with the environment and others. Recognising emotional entrainment as a core feature of social life invites a shift toward more integrated models of psychology, sociology, and anthropology that foreground the body's role in shaping collective consciousness.

Practically, insights into emotional entrainment inform a range of fields—from the design of public spaces that encourage positive social interaction, to therapeutic practices employing group movement for trauma recovery, to political organising strategies that mobilise affect through embodied rituals. For instance, community dance programs have been used to repair social fractures in post-conflict zones by fostering embodied empathy and shared emotional experiences. Similarly, mindful movement workshops leverage synchronized breathing and gestures to enhance group cohesion and emotional regulation among participants with mental health challenges.

Ultimately, the study of contagious motion and contagious emotion illuminates the profound ways in which human beings are wired to move and feel together. It calls attention to the body as a medium through which social bonds are forged and collective moods are shaped, revealing movement not simply as physical activity but as a language of connection and a generator of shared meaning. As we navigate increasingly fragmented societies, recognising and cultivating emotional entrainment offers a pathway toward rebuilding empathy, solidarity, and collective wellbeing through the simple, ancient act of moving in harmony.

Movement as Language of Belonging

From the ritualised clapping of sports fans to the synchronized chants of religious congregations, shared movement is a profound medium through which humans communicate, connect, and cultivate belonging. This somatic language operates beneath and alongside spoken words, transcending linguistic barriers to evoke a visceral sense of unity. Across cultures and contexts, the synchrony of bodies—marching, dancing, gesturing—creates bonds that often run deeper than verbal dialogue, reflecting an ancient, embodied mode of sociality embedded in our evolutionary heritage.

At the heart of this phenomenon lies the neurobiological substrate of *mirror neurons*, a system that underpins our capacity for imitation, empathy, and social learning. Discovered in primates and later identified in humans, mirror neurons fire both when we perform an action and when we observe others performing the same action. This mirroring facilitates a somatic resonance that blurs the boundaries between self and other, enabling us to internalise and share emotional states through observed movement. For example, the subtle mimicry of posture or facial expression in everyday interactions fosters rapport and trust, while more overt coordinated actions amplify group cohesion and collective identity.

The role of mimicry extends beyond unconscious mirroring to encompass intentional synchronization, often cultivated in group settings. Coordinated movement—whether in team sports, dance ensembles, or military drills—requires attunement not only to one's own body but to the rhythm and flow of others. This dynamic coordination produces *interpersonal synchrony*, a state in which individuals' movements become temporally aligned, enhancing feelings of connectedness and cooperation. Experimental studies have shown that participants engaged in synchronous activities report increased affiliation, altruism, and social bonding, effects that persist beyond the immediate context. This highlights how movement is a fundamental social glue, forging relationships through embodied dialogue.

Sports teams exemplify the power of movement as a language of belonging. The rituals surrounding training, warm-ups, and gameplay—high-fives, chants, tactical formations—encode shared meaning and reinforce a collective identity. These practices are not merely performative; they generate a somatic attunement that undergirds teamwork, enabling members to anticipate and respond to each other's actions seamlessly. The embodied synchrony within a team fosters a sense of "we-ness" that transcends individual differences, aligning players around common goals and shared emotional experiences.

Religious and spiritual rituals similarly harness the communicative potency of shared movement. Ceremonial dances, processions, and collective postures serve to enact and embody communal values and narratives. The repetitive, rhythmic nature of these movements often induces altered states of consciousness, facilitating transcendence and group cohesion. Anthropological research reveals that such embodied practices function as *embodied metaphors*, translating abstract spiritual concepts into tangible, lived experience. The movement itself becomes a sacred language, articulating belonging not only to a community but to a cosmological order.

While the unifying effects of shared movement are compelling, they also raise questions about individual autonomy and social conformity. Coordinated motion can simultaneously foster inclusion and exclusion, delineating who belongs and who does not. The ritualised aspects of movement can impose normative behaviours that suppress dissent or diversity, underscoring the ambivalence inherent in embodied sociality. Critical perspectives urge us to consider how movement practices may reinforce power structures, social hierarchies, or cultural homogenisation, prompting reflection on the ethics of embodied belonging.

Contemporary applications further illuminate the multifaceted role of movement in social connection. Therapeutic approaches such as dance/movement therapy utilise synchrony and mimicry to rebuild relational trust and self-awareness in clinical populations. Corporate team-building exercises often incorporate coordinated activities to enhance collaboration and morale. Even digital interfaces now explore embodied synchrony through virtual reality and motion capture technologies, seeking to replicate the affective bonds formed through physical co-presence. These developments attest to the enduring relevance of movement as a primary social language.

Philosophically, recognising movement as a language of belonging challenges dominant Western paradigms privileging rational discourse as the apex of communication. Instead, it foregrounds embodied experience as foundational to meaning-making and sociality. This perspective resonates with phenomenological and embodied cognition theories, which posit that our being-in-the-world is constituted through sensorimotor engagement rather than abstract cognition alone. Movement, therefore, is not ancillary but central to how we understand ourselves in relation to others.

Ultimately, exploring movement as a language of belonging invites a renewed appreciation of the body's role in shaping social life. It reveals how our gestures, rhythms, and coordinated actions weave the fabric of human connection, creating shared emotional landscapes and collective identities. By attuning to this embodied discourse, individuals and communities can cultivate deeper empathy, more authentic collaboration, and richer forms of belonging that transcend words. This chapter illuminates a dimension of human experience that is as vital as it is often overlooked—the silent, powerful language of moving together.

Bodies in Resistance

The body has long served as both a site of oppression and a powerful instrument of resistance. In contexts where voices are silenced, movements surveilled, and identities marginalised, embodied action emerges as a vital form of political speech—an eloquent, nonverbal assertion of agency and identity. From the marchers of the civil rights era to the practitioners of Afro-Brazilian Capoeira, bodies in motion have enacted defiance, forged solidarity, and rewritten narratives imposed by dominant power structures. This embodied resistance challenges conventional notions of protest as purely verbal or ideological, revealing how motion itself can disrupt, reclaim, and transform.

Historically, social and political movements have harnessed the visceral power of collective movement to contest injustice and galvanise communities. The civil rights marches of the 1960s in the United States provide a seminal example. Marchers deliberately occupied public space, their coordinated steps an audible and visible claim to rights denied. The embodied act of walking together signified unity and resolve, transforming the physical act of movement into a potent symbol of resistance. Scholars such as Heather Ann Thompson have highlighted how these marches were not only political demonstrations but also embodied performances that communicated dignity, defiance, and hope. The simple synchrony of footfalls became a drumbeat of social change, echoing beyond the streets into the cultural and legislative fabric of the nation.

Beyond marches, embodied resistance takes myriad cultural forms. Capoeira, the Afro-Brazilian martial art blending dance, acrobatics, and music, originated among enslaved Africans as a covert form of self-defence and cultural preservation under colonial repression. Its fluid, deceptive movements masked a deeper political meaning—a bodily language encoding survival, resilience, and communal identity. As historian Thomas J. Desch-Obi notes, Capoeira's circular formations and rhythmic interplay serve both as physical resistance and as a challenge to colonial hierarchies. The embodied dialogue within the roda (circle) fosters not only skill but a shared sense of history and empowerment. Here, motion becomes a repository of memory and a medium for reclaiming agency when speech was prohibited.

Similar dynamics unfold in other oppressed communities. Indigenous dance rituals, for example, have long functioned as acts of cultural resistance, preserving languages, cosmologies, and social bonds in the face of colonial erasure. The embodied repetition of ancestral movements asserts continuity and belonging, challenging narratives of disappearance or assimilation. Contemporary movements for Indigenous rights frequently incorporate such embodied practices to reclaim sovereignty and articulate collective grief or hope. This intersection of body and politics underscores how movement transcends individual expression to enact communal resilience and contestation.

The neuroscientific concept of *embodied cognition* sheds light on why movement serves as such an effective mode of resistance. Our brains do not process thought and emotion as detached from bodily states; instead, cognition is deeply intertwined with sensorimotor experience. Movements—whether marching, dancing, or gesturing—activate neural circuits that reinforce emotional and social bonds, generating affective states aligned with collective purpose. This neurological basis for embodied resistance helps explain why coordinated physical action can mobilise solidarity more profoundly than verbal appeals alone.

Yet embodied resistance also faces challenges and complexities. States of surveillance, criminalisation, or cultural appropriation can undermine or distort the meanings of movement-based practices. For instance, state responses to protest often seek to disrupt embodied solidarity through policing tactics aimed at breaking up groups or delegitimising their physical presence. Similarly, cultural forms like Capoeira risk commodification when divorced from their historical contexts, raising questions about authenticity and cultural sovereignty. These tensions highlight the need for critical engagement with the ethical dimensions of embodied political expression.

Contemporary social movements continue to innovate embodied resistance in response to shifting political landscapes. The Black Lives Matter protests, climate marches, and feminist demonstrations worldwide employ choreographed marches, die-ins, and rhythmic clapping to communicate urgency and unity. Digital activism, while primarily virtual, often incorporates embodied elements through viral dance challenges or coordinated physical gatherings, blending corporeal presence with mediated communication. This hybridisation signals the ongoing evolution of bodies in resistance within globalised, digitised societies.

Therapeutically, recognising the political power of embodied resistance informs trauma-informed practices that empower marginalised individuals to reclaim agency through movement. Dance and somatic therapies enable survivors of violence or displacement to access and express emotions beyond language, fostering healing grounded in embodied autonomy. These approaches affirm that resistance is not solely external protest but also internal reclamation of selfhood through bodily presence.

Philosophically, the concept of bodies in resistance disrupts Cartesian dualisms separating mind and body, thought and action, individual and society. It demands a holistic understanding of politics as enacted through embodied being-in-the-world. This perspective aligns with feminist and postcolonial theories emphasising the situated, material realities of oppression and the embodied strategies of contestation. Recognising the body as a site of both subjugation and insurgency deepens our grasp of power dynamics and the possibilities for transformation.

Ultimately, exploring bodies in resistance reveals movement as a language of emancipation—a form of political speech that transcends words and engages the full sensorimotor self. It calls attention to the profound ways in which embodied action can disrupt dominant narratives, forge collective identities, and open spaces for justice. As societies confront ongoing struggles for equity and recognition, acknowledging and honouring the political significance of moving bodies remains essential to understanding how change unfolds not only in minds but in the very motion of human life.

Dancing Together, Healing Together

Healing is rarely an individual endeavour. Across cultures and throughout history, communal movement has functioned as a profound channel for emotional reconciliation and collective restoration. The shared experience of embodied rituals—be it through dance, drumming, or rhythmic gestures—enables groups to process trauma, express grief, and reaffirm bonds beyond what language alone can convey. This somatic communal healing reveals the body not just as a vessel for personal health, but as a site where collective wounds are tended, social cohesion restored, and emotional landscapes rebalanced.

In many African societies, for example, grief is not an isolated burden but a communal event marked by elaborate rituals involving dance and drumming. These practices are far from mere cultural artefacts; they are dynamic, lived expressions of psychological and social repair. The rhythms of the drum serve as temporal anchors, guiding bodies into synchrony and emotional resonance. As participants move together, they engage in what ethnomusicologist John Blacking termed "musical entrainment," a physiological and psychological phenomenon that fosters empathy and mutual attunement. This shared rhythm creates a safe container for the expression of sorrow and remembrance, transforming personal loss into a collective act of witnessing and validation.

Indigenous drumming circles offer another striking example of embodied healing as community practice. In various Indigenous North American cultures, drumming is a sacred act that connects individuals to their ancestors, the land, and one another. The repetitive, grounding beat induces altered states of consciousness, facilitating emotional release and spiritual connection. Participants report feelings of unity, renewal, and a deepened sense of belonging—effects corroborated by contemporary psychophysiological research demonstrating reduced stress markers and enhanced emotional regulation following such ceremonies. These embodied practices affirm that healing extends beyond cognitive processing, reaching into the somatic and relational domains.

The neuroscience behind these communal movements underscores their transformative potential. Studies on mirror neurons reveal that observing and synchronising with others' movements activates neural circuits associated with empathy and social bonding. This embodied mimicry supports the concept of "emotional contagion," where feelings spread through groups not by words but through shared physicality. Such mechanisms explain why coordinated group movement can dissolve barriers, reduce feelings of isolation, and foster collective resilience in the face of adversity.

Beyond ritualistic contexts, contemporary somatic therapies integrate community-based movement to address trauma and emotional dysregulation. Modalities like Ecstatic Dance and Trauma

Releasing Exercises (TRE) harness group dynamics to facilitate nonverbal expression and somatic discharge. By moving together in unstructured yet intentional ways, participants unlock deeply held tensions and reconnect fragmented bodily awareness. Facilitators often emphasise the importance of attuned witnessing—being fully present with others' movements and emotional states—as a cornerstone of healing. This relational somatic attention cultivates safety and nurtures the restorative power of embodied empathy.

However, the politics of embodied healing warrant critical scrutiny. Practices rooted in Indigenous or traditional knowledge risk appropriation or dilution when removed from their cultural and ethical contexts. The commodification of "sacred" movement forms within wellness industries sometimes strips them of their communal and reparative functions, reducing them to mere physical exercise or entertainment. Respecting the provenance and integrity of these practices requires not only acknowledgment but ongoing engagement with the communities from which they originate, ensuring that healing remains collective, reciprocal, and just.

Moreover, the efficacy of somatic community healing challenges Western paradigms that prioritise verbal psychotherapy and individualism. Western psychological frameworks often struggle to address the embodied, relational dimensions of trauma and grief. Incorporating communal movement as a therapeutic resource demands an epistemological shift toward valuing nonverbal, embodied knowledge and the social embeddedness of healing. This approach aligns with intersectional understandings of health that consider how cultural, historical, and social factors shape emotional experience and recovery.

Philosophically, collective somatic practices enact a form of "body politic" where the personal and political interlace through movement. They assert that bodies, especially those marginalised or traumatised, carry histories that cannot be resolved solely through cognition or speech. By coming together in shared motion, communities rewrite narratives of pain and fragmentation into stories of resilience and reconnection. This embodied agency expands the horizons of healing beyond the individual psyche into the realm of social transformation.

In the context of global crises—whether pandemics, racial injustice, or environmental disasters—the need for embodied collective healing has become increasingly urgent. Social distancing and isolation have underscored the essential human need for physical presence and shared rhythm. Virtual adaptations of group movement practices have attempted to bridge these gaps, highlighting the adaptability and necessity of communal embodiment even when physical proximity is limited. Such innovations affirm the timeless relevance of dancing and moving together as a source of solace, strength, and shared humanity.

Ultimately, "dancing together, healing together" is more than a poetic phrase; it is an empirical and lived truth. The choreography of communal movement invites us to reclaim the body as a site of emotional reconciliation and social connection. It calls on us to recognise that healing emerges not only through solitary reflection but through embodied, collective expression—where the rhythm of many hearts and feet can mend what solitude fractures. Through these shared somatic languages, communities rediscover their capacity to bear witness, to grieve, and ultimately, to heal in concert.

Chapter 8
Ritual, Myth, and the Sacred Body

The pulse of ancient ritual once carried human life with a cadence that was both sacred and visceral, entwining flesh and spirit in moments of ecstatic communion. The frenzied dances of Dionysian initiates, the solemn pacing of pilgrims tracing sanctified routes—such acts of embodied devotion were not mere spectacles but vehicles of psychic renewal and spiritual transformation. Their erosion in modernity has left a peculiar vacancy, a kind of spiritual restlessness marked by alienation and an uneasy hunger for depth. This chapter proposes a return of sorts: not a nostalgic imitation of the past, but a reimagining of the body as consecrated ground, a site where myth, ritual, and psyche intersect. It makes the case for rekindling personal and communal rites of movement—acts not of ornament but of necessity—for meaning, balance, and psychic repair in a culture that often reduces the body to instrument or ornament.

Consider the legacy. In ancient Greece, Dionysian rites unfolded in waves of drumming, stamping, spinning—states where ego dissolved, and chaos braided with order. Here participants slipped into altered consciousness, allowing the unconscious to surge forward in forms unmediated by reason. What felt to outsiders like indulgent abandon was, in truth, a portal into depths of psyche and spirit. Neuroscience now begins to explain what ancient practice intuited: ritualised ecstasy reshapes neural networks governing emotion, identity, and integration. The irony is plain—while our ancestors danced their way into wholeness, we, shaped by the industrial and digital age, find ourselves fragmented, seated, restless, and profoundly hungry for connection.

Jungian psychology provides a further bridge. Archetypes—those universal images lodged in the collective unconscious—do not live only in dream and symbol; they breathe in movement. The firm advance of the Warrior, the unguarded skip of the Child, the weighted sway of the Crone—each gesture summons a psychic force. When enacted with intention, such movements are not performance but dialogue, a way of drawing shadow into light, of coaxing creativity from silence. Ritual theatre, martial arts, dance:

these are not diversions but languages through which psyche converses with soma, reshaping the inner landscape.

The pilgrimage, too, offers a template for embodied transformation. The Camino de Santiago, the Hajj—such journeys are not reducible to geography. Each step is a shedding, each mile a quiet dismantling of self, making room for renewal. The rhythm of walking, repeated over days or weeks, lulls the mind into meditation, inviting grief to surface, clarity to settle. Testimonies abound of pilgrims who return altered—lighter, more whole, carrying an orientation to life that no classroom or sermon could impart. Movement across land becomes an outer mirror of inner metamorphosis, proving again that transformation is never purely mental but carved through the body.

But the sacred need not always wear the robes of grand tradition. It can flicker in smaller gestures: a breath taken deliberately, a stretch offered in reverence, the slow rhythm of a mindful walk between ordinary tasks. These micro-rituals are antidotes to mechanised life, sanctifying the mundane and reminding us that transcendence hides within reach. They are not trivial embellishments but practices that root mood, strengthen resilience, and call the sacred into daily life—small anchors against the drift of alienation.

Still, we must tread carefully. To borrow from ancestral rituals without context risks hollow imitation, even appropriation. Yet to ignore their wisdom altogether is to surrender a vital inheritance. The challenge, then, is to craft rituals attuned to contemporary existence—gestures informed by myth and archetype but grounded in the specificity of one's own life and community. Innovation and tradition need not be adversaries; together they can breathe new life into the old truth that the body is both threshold and temple.

What emerges, finally, is a vision of ritual, myth, and the sacred body as inseparable strands of a holistic psychology. To move with reverence is to acknowledge that the body is not merely mechanical but mythic, not simply functional but alive with significance. This chapter extends an invitation: to rediscover the body as an agent of meaning, a participant in the making of self and society, and to shape rituals—ancient or invented—that restore us to our own depths. In this light, movement ceases to be ordinary exercise. It becomes prayer, resistance, remembrance. It becomes, quite simply, a way home.

Mythic Movement: From Dionysus to Digital Detox

The human body has long been a vessel of sacred expression, where movement transcends mere physicality to become a conduit of ecstasy, connection, and meaning. In ancient societies, rituals of embodied ecstasy—often communal, rhythmic, and trance-inducing—served as essential cultural practices that integrated mind, body, and spirit. The Dionysian rites of classical Greece, for example, were not merely celebratory dances but profound ceremonies that dissolved the boundaries between the self and the divine, enabling participants to access a collective unconsciousness and release pent-up emotional and spiritual tensions. These embodied rituals were central to communal cohesion and individual psychological renewal, offering a cyclical pattern of descent and ascent, chaos and order, suffering and joy. Yet, as modernity has progressed, these ritualistic movements have largely vanished from everyday life, leaving a void that manifests as a pervasive spiritual malaise and disconnection from the body's deeper wisdom.

The decline of ritualized embodied ecstasy is not accidental but intricately tied to the rise of rationalism, industrialisation, and the fragmentation of communal life. The mechanisation of labour and the rise of individualism relegated the body to a mere tool of productivity rather than a sacred medium of expression. Simultaneously, the rise of secularism and scientific reductionism dismissed ecstatic movement as superstition or irrational indulgence. This historical shift has left contemporary society grappling with symptoms of this disembodiment: chronic stress, alienation, and a sense of existential emptiness that no amount of intellectual or technological advancement seems able to alleviate. Neuroscientific studies corroborate that the lack of rhythmic, communal movement impairs emotional regulation and social bonding, pointing to an embodied deficit at the heart of modern psychological distress.

In recent decades, however, a growing movement toward "digital detox" and embodied practices signals an implicit recognition of what has been lost. The return to body-centred rituals—whether through ecstatic dance festivals, yoga, or somatic therapies—represents an attempt to re-engage the body's capacity for sacred, transformative experience. Unlike the Dionysian rites, these contemporary practices are often solitary or highly individualised, reflecting modern values of personal autonomy. Yet, they share a common thread: an acknowledgement that movement, when consciously embodied, functions as a portal to altered states of consciousness, healing, and reconnection with something larger than the self.

Reinventing personal rituals of movement in the modern context requires both a reclamation and an innovation. It demands an understanding of the symbolic and psychological dimensions of movement, alongside a practical recognition of contemporary lifestyles and sensibilities. Ritual scholar Catherine Bell emphasises that rituals are not static relics but dynamic performances that must adapt to the needs of their practitioners. Thus, personal rituals might integrate elements of ancient ecstasy with mindfulness, creativity, and community engagement, blending spontaneity with intention. For instance, the practice of "free dance" within therapeutic or communal settings can evoke a state akin to Dionysian ecstasy, while also offering a safe container for emotional exploration and expression.

Moreover, the neuroscientific concept of neuroplasticity provides a biological framework for understanding how ritualised movement can rewire patterns of brain function related to mood, trauma, and identity. Repeated engagement in embodied rituals fosters integration between limbic structures (emotion centres) and prefrontal regions (executive functions), enhancing emotional resilience and cognitive flexibility. This evidence underscores that ritual movement is not merely symbolic but fundamentally reparative, addressing the embodied scars left by disconnection and cultural neglect.

At the same time, the revival of ritualized movement must remain critically aware of cultural appropriation and the ethical complexities of transplanting sacred practices across contexts. The contemporary embrace of ecstatic dance and indigenous movement traditions risks diluting or commodifying practices that carry profound cultural and spiritual significance. Ethical reinvention involves respectful study, collaboration with originating communities, and an openness to diverse expressions rather than homogenised trends. This approach honours the multiplicity of ways bodies have been—and continue to be—moved by myth and spirit.

The embodied ecstasies of the past also remind us that movement rituals are inherently political acts. In their capacity to dissolve boundaries, they disrupt hierarchical and normative structures, creating liminal spaces for liberation and transformation. The absence of such communal, transformative movement in mainstream culture can thus be understood as a form of social control, limiting access to the collective power of the body. Personal rituals, then, become not only acts of healing but subtle forms of resistance, reclaiming agency over one's body and psyche.

In sum, the arc from Dionysus to digital detox traces a profound cultural shift and the ongoing human yearning to restore sacred connection through movement. This chapter invites readers to rediscover movement as a language of myth and spirit, to invent rituals that resonate personally and communally, and to engage with the body as a living archive of transformation. It positions embodied ecstasy not as an indulgence but as an essential, foundational practice for psychological and spiritual wellbeing. Through thoughtful reinvention of ritual, the body can once again become a temple—alive with meaning, rhythm, and transcendence in the contemporary world.

The Psyche Dances

The human psyche, with its labyrinthine depths and multifaceted layers, often defies direct articulation. Carl Gustav Jung, the seminal figure in analytical psychology, proposed that beneath our conscious awareness lies a rich terrain of archetypes—universal, primordial images and motifs that shape our inner world and behaviour. These archetypes, far from being mere abstractions, manifest vividly through symbols, dreams, myths, and crucially, through the body's movement. In the realm of embodied practice, the psyche dances. Movement becomes an expressive language through which these archetypes are not only encountered but experienced viscerally, opening portals to unconscious knowledge and transformation. This subchapter explores how engaging with archetypal movement—embodying figures such as the Warrior, the Child, or the Crone—can deepen our psychological insight, enliven creativity, and foster integration of fragmented parts of the self.

Jung's theory of archetypes underscores their role as collective psychic structures inherited across generations. Unlike personal memories or learned behaviours, archetypes resonate universally, appearing in myths and rituals worldwide. Movement, as a non-verbal mode of expression, provides a direct conduit to these archetypes, bypassing intellectual filters and facilitating embodied encounters with the unconscious. When we move as the Warrior, for example, we tap into the archetype's qualities of strength, courage, and assertion. This is not a mere role-play but an enactment that can awaken dormant inner resources, realigning the individual with a vital aspect of their psyche. Similarly, the Child archetype, characterised by innocence, spontaneity, and curiosity, can be embodied through playful, expansive gestures that invite renewal and creative openness. The Crone, symbolising wisdom, transformation, and acceptance of mortality, can emerge in slow, grounded, and deliberate movements that honour the body's aging and evolving nature.

The transformative potential of archetypal movement has found practical application across therapeutic and artistic domains. Dance therapy, for instance, frequently draws on Jungian principles, guiding participants to explore archetypal motifs through improvisation and somatic inquiry. Case studies illustrate how clients can access repressed emotions, integrate shadow aspects, and reclaim lost parts of themselves by embodying archetypes. In performance psychology, actors and dancers employ archetypal movement to enrich character development, deepen emotional truth, and create resonant narratives that engage audiences on unconscious levels. This dual therapeutic and artistic application reveals the profound versatility of archetypal embodiment as both self-exploration and communicative act.

Engagement with archetypal movement also challenges contemporary Western dualisms that separate mind and body, rationality and emotion, conscious and unconscious. Jung himself viewed the psyche as fundamentally embodied, rejecting purely cerebral models of consciousness. Modern somatic psychology echoes this, positing that the body stores implicit memories and unconscious material. Movement thus becomes a form of 'psychic dialogue'—a dynamic interplay where the individual listens to the body's signals and responds creatively. This dialogic process not only unveils archetypal energies but also allows for their conscious integration, reducing fragmentation and fostering wholeness. Importantly, archetypal movement resists reduction to technique or exercise; it is a poetic and spiritual practice that honours mystery, paradox, and the non-linear nature of psychic transformation.

Nevertheless, working with archetypes through movement entails conceptual tensions and ethical considerations. Archetypes, while universal, are culturally inflected and can be misappropriated or stereotyped if engaged superficially. For example, the Warrior archetype may be narrowly interpreted as aggression or dominance, overlooking its protective and honourable dimensions. Similarly, embodying the Crone requires sensitivity to gendered and ageist biases that may distort its meaning. Practitioners must therefore cultivate nuanced, respectful approaches that foreground personal resonance and cultural context. Reflexivity and openness to complexity safeguard against simplistic caricatures and ensure that archetypal work remains a source of empowerment rather than confinement.

From a neuroscientific perspective, embodied archetypal engagement aligns with findings on mirror neurons and embodied cognition, which reveal how observing or enacting movements associated with emotional states activates corresponding neural circuits. This biological grounding lends credence to the idea that archetypal movement can influence emotional regulation, memory reconsolidation, and neural plasticity. It suggests that through repeated, intentional movement patterns that evoke archetypal qualities, individuals may recondition habitual responses and access adaptive psychic states. This convergence of psychological theory, embodied practice, and neuroscience points to a fertile interdisciplinary frontier for further research and application.

In contemporary cultural contexts marked by disconnection and over-intellectualisation, archetypal movement offers a route back to embodied presence and imaginative engagement with the unconscious. It invites individuals to rediscover movement not merely as physical activity but as a symbolic, integrative language that bridges inner and outer worlds. Through ritualised enactments of archetypes, people can confront shadow material, summon latent strengths, and participate in a collective heritage of myth and symbol. Such practices resonate deeply with those seeking psychological depth, creative inspiration, and spiritual nourishment in a fragmented modern landscape.

Ultimately, the psyche dances because it is alive, restless, and yearning for expression beyond words. Embodying archetypes through movement is not a return to mythic nostalgia but a vital, living practice of psychological alchemy—transforming raw instinct and unconscious material into conscious wholeness. This chapter offers readers both theoretical foundations and practical pathways to engage the dance of the psyche, encouraging an embodied dialogue with the timeless figures that dwell within us all. It is an invitation to move with intention, openness, and reverence into the deep currents of the self.

Pilgrimage and the Psychology of Journeying

The act of pilgrimage, particularly walking pilgrimages such as the Camino de Santiago or the Hajj, holds a powerful place in both cultural history and the psychology of transformation. These journeys extend far beyond physical travel; they embody profound metaphors for the inner movement of the self. The physical act of moving through diverse terrains and stages mirrors psychological processes of change, challenge, and renewal. Far from a mere religious or cultural custom, pilgrimage can be understood as a living symbol of psychological journeying—an embodied rite of passage that enacts the transformation of identity, meaning, and consciousness through the movement of the body in space. This subchapter explores the multilayered dynamics of walking pilgrimages as symbolic and somatic processes, illuminating how the external journey maps onto inner transformation.

At its core, pilgrimage involves a deliberate displacement from familiar surroundings into liminal space, a threshold that invites transition. The physical challenge of the walk—enduring fatigue, discomfort, and uncertainty—acts as a catalyst for psychological shifts. The slow rhythm of footsteps over days or weeks fosters a deepened attentiveness to the present moment and bodily sensations, cultivating a heightened self-awareness often lacking in hurried modern life. This embodied awareness opens a space for confronting unresolved internal conflicts, integrating disparate aspects of the psyche, and reframing personal narratives. The external pilgrimage route, therefore, becomes a metaphorical canvas on which the pilgrim enacts processes of grief, hope, transformation, and surrender.

The Camino de Santiago, one of the most studied contemporary pilgrimage routes, exemplifies these dynamics. Originally a medieval Christian pilgrimage to the shrine of Saint James in northwestern Spain, the Camino today attracts diverse participants, including those seeking spiritual renewal, psychological healing, or a break from the digital world's relentless pace. Empirical studies have documented the Camino's psychological impact, highlighting enhanced wellbeing, increased mindfulness, and a sense of profound connection with self and others among pilgrims. The process of moving sequentially through stages—physically marked by milestones and symbolically by ritual acts such as collecting stamps or attending communal meals—facilitates a narrative restructuring that supports identity growth and emotional resolution.

Similarly, the Hajj pilgrimage to Mecca, a central pillar of Islamic practice, encapsulates a potent interplay of collective ritual and individual transformation. The precise movements, prescribed rites, and cyclical repetitions of the Hajj enact a dissolution of the ego-self and an experience of unity with the divine and the global Muslim community. Psychologically, this surrender of individual boundaries through coordinated movement resonates with theories of self-transcendence and peak experience. The embodiment of ritual gestures—circling the Kaaba, walking between Safa and Marwah—

can be understood as somatic anchors for spiritual and psychic transformation, anchoring transcendent states in bodily memory.

These pilgrimage traditions also highlight the essential role of rhythm and repetition in fostering transformation. Repeated movement patterns create a trance-like state that dissolves habitual thought patterns and facilitates access to unconscious material. The interplay of solitude and communal interaction along pilgrimage routes further intensifies emotional processing and the development of empathy and social connectedness. Such features suggest that pilgrimage is not only an individual psychological event but a deeply social process that shapes collective identity and cultural memory.

From a psychological perspective, pilgrimage can be situated within the framework of ritual and rite of passage theories articulated by scholars such as Arnold van Gennep and Victor Turner. The stages of separation, liminality, and reintegration align with the physical and symbolic phases of pilgrimage. Liminality—the ambiguous, betwixt-and-between state during the journey—is a crucible for transformation, where old identities dissolve, and new possibilities emerge. Movement through space becomes a somatic enactment of this threshold state, allowing for experiential learning and the emergence of novel ways of being.

Contemporary psychological research also intersects with embodied cognition theories, which propose that bodily states influence mental and emotional processes. Walking pilgrimages engage the body's sensorimotor systems in ways that reshape cognition and affect. The kinaesthetic intelligence cultivated through sustained walking facilitates a grounded presence and embodied mindfulness, reducing rumination and promoting emotional regulation. This neuropsychological lens enriches our understanding of how pilgrimage movement serves as a mechanism for healing and growth.

However, pilgrimage's metaphorical power extends beyond spiritual or therapeutic realms. It raises critical questions about privilege, access, and cultural appropriation. Pilgrimage, historically embedded in specific religious and cultural contexts, is increasingly commodified in the global wellness industry. The transformation of pilgrimage into tourism risks diluting its symbolic potency and overlooks the socio-political dimensions of these journeys. An ethically informed engagement with pilgrimage as psychological metaphor requires attentiveness to these tensions and a respect for the traditions from which these embodied practices emerge.

For the contemporary seeker, pilgrimage need not be confined to canonical routes or religious frameworks. Personal rituals of journeying—whether walking through urban landscapes, wilderness treks, or slow, intentional movement in daily life—can enact similar psychodynamic processes. The essential ingredients remain: deliberate movement through space, openness to liminal experience, and receptivity to symbolic meaning. These practices offer a pathway to counteract modern disembodiment and fragmentation, reconnecting body and psyche through the art of moving with intention.

Ultimately, pilgrimage as a psychology of journeying invites us to reconsider movement not as mere locomotion but as a deeply symbolic, transformative act. The body's traversal across physical terrain becomes a mirror of inner passage, an external narrative that catalyses internal change. This embodied metaphor enriches our understanding of movement's potential to shape identity, meaning, and healing, bridging ancient ritual with contemporary psychological insight. As we step forward, we embody not only physical progression but a profound engagement with the unfolding story of self.

Creating Sacred Space in the Everyday

Transforming ordinary movement into an act of sacred attention offers a profound antidote to the disconnection and hurriedness of contemporary life. In a culture dominated by multitasking and digital distractions, the simple act of walking or stretching risks becoming a mechanical routine devoid of meaning. Yet, embedded within these everyday motions lies an untapped potential to cultivate presence, elevate mood, and anchor a deeper sense of self. This subchapter unpacks how seemingly mundane physical acts can be consciously reframed as sacred practices—rituals that infuse ordinary movement with intentionality, reverence, and psychological nourishment.

The notion of creating sacred space in daily life is often relegated to designated places or formal ceremonies. However, a growing body of research and embodied philosophy reveals that sacredness is less about location and more about quality of attention. Drawing on mindfulness principles, phenomenology, and somatic psychology, this approach emphasises *how* we move rather than *what* we do. When movement is performed with focused awareness, attuned to subtle bodily sensations and emotional currents, it becomes a bridge between the external and internal worlds—a dialogue with the self that enriches both.

Real-world examples illustrate this transformation vividly. Consider the mindful walking practice adopted by many spiritual traditions: rather than rushing from one point to another, practitioners slow their gait to feel each footfall, synchronise breath with movement, and observe the surrounding environment with openness and gratitude. In these moments, a simple walk transcends transportation and becomes a meditation in motion. Likewise, restorative yoga sequences emphasise slow, deliberate stretching paired with breath awareness, inviting practitioners to explore tension and release while cultivating acceptance and self-compassion. Scientific studies corroborate the benefits of such embodied practices, linking mindful movement with reduced anxiety, enhanced mood regulation, and improved interoceptive awareness—the ability to perceive internal bodily states.

At the heart of creating sacred movement lies the concept of *intention.* Unlike habitual or goal-oriented exercise, sacred movement begins with setting an intention to engage fully with the present moment and honour the body's lived experience. This conscious framing alters the neurophysiological landscape, activating parasympathetic pathways associated with relaxation and emotional regulation. Intentionality also reshapes narrative meaning: a stretch is no longer a mere physical act but a gesture of kindness towards oneself; a walk becomes a ritual of grounding and connection with the earth. This shift from function to meaning expands movement's capacity to transform mood and foster psychological integration.

Yet, cultivating sacred space in everyday movement is not without conceptual tensions. Western utilitarian frameworks often privilege productivity and measurable outcomes, potentially conflicting with the slow, receptive stance sacred movement requires. Moreover, there is a risk of spiritual bypass—using ritualised movement to escape rather than engage with difficult emotions. Addressing these complexities demands an ethical and nuanced approach, emphasising emotional honesty alongside reverence. Facilitators and individuals alike must hold space for vulnerability, allowing movement to evoke and process a spectrum of feelings rather than enforcing a prescribed 'positive' affect.

Technological advances and urban living further complicate access to sacred movement. The bombardment of sensory stimuli and sedentary lifestyles challenge the ability to attune inwardly. Yet, paradoxically, technology can also support sacred movement when harnessed thoughtfully. Digital platforms now offer guided somatic practices, virtual meditation walks, and biofeedback tools that encourage embodied awareness. The key lies in integrating these resources without losing touch with the body's innate wisdom and the organic rhythm of natural environments.

The transformative potential of creating sacred space in the everyday extends into social and cultural realms as well. Communal practices such as circle dances, drum circles, and collective yoga sessions illustrate how shared intentional movement fosters belonging and collective healing. These embodied gatherings reconnect participants with ancestral traditions and communal narratives, counteracting social fragmentation. In such contexts, sacred movement becomes a form of cultural memory and a catalyst for social cohesion.

Practical strategies for cultivating sacred movement can be incorporated seamlessly into daily routines. Simple acts such as pausing before standing to take a deep breath, performing a short sequence of mindful stretches upon waking, or dedicating attention to the sensations of walking to the mailbox invite moments of ritualised presence. Over time, these micro-practices accumulate, transforming mundane movement into sustained pathways of self-awareness and emotional balance.

Philosophically, creating sacred space in everyday movement challenges dualistic mind-body paradigms by insisting on the unity of embodied experience. Movement becomes a language through which the psyche speaks and listens, an ongoing negotiation between conscious intention and unconscious impulse. This perspective aligns with contemporary theories in embodied cognition, somatic psychotherapy, and contemplative traditions, offering a comprehensive framework for understanding movement as a vital source of meaning and psychological resilience.

Ultimately, the act of infusing ordinary movement with sacred attention reclaims the body as a site of wisdom and reverence. It invites a radical reorientation from disembodied doing to embodied being, from fragmented distraction to integrated presence. By weaving intention, mindfulness, and reverence into the fabric of everyday movement, individuals can access profound shifts in mood, self-connection, and wellbeing. This transformation not only enriches personal life but also cultivates a more mindful and compassionate culture—one step, one breath, one stretch at a time.

Chapter 9
Designing a Movement Practice for Emotional Integration

The dominant story told about exercise tends to cast movement as a prescription: a set of tasks designed to correct, improve, or measure the body's output—steps counted, calories burned, kilos lifted. Useful, perhaps, in some contexts, but this framing conceals a deeper reality. Movement is not merely mechanical labour; it is relational, expressive, alive. Each gesture links us to our emotions, our history, our very sense of who we are. This chapter invites the reader to dismantle the sterile view of exercise as duty and to reimagine movement as ritual—an act whose purpose lies less in efficiency than in emotional integration, less in metrics than in meaning.

To do so requires a redefinition of what it means to 'exercise.' No longer is it a task to check off, nor a performance perfected under watchful eyes. Instead, it becomes dialogue—one shaped by mood, trauma, resilience, even tenderness. Affective neuroscience and somatic psychology have long suggested that the body is not a mute carrier of feeling but an active participant in its processing. Emotions are shaped, shifted, sometimes resolved through patterns of movement. In practical terms, this suggests a practice that bends to the contours of inner life rather than forcing itself upon them—fluid, responsive, attuned.

Within this vision, the chapter introduces what it calls mood-based movement maps. Think of them not as prescriptive remedies but as invitations. Swimming, with its encompassing element, lends itself to grief's release. Boxing, sharp and cathartic, gives anger a channel. Tai chi offers meditative flow; walking grounds the restless. The map does not dictate what must be done but opens paths of exploration, encouraging each person to notice which modalities harmonise with their present state and to follow that resonance with patience and self-compassion.

Equally important are the feedback loops one learns to cultivate. This is less technical than it sounds: it is the act of listening—before, during, after. How does the body feel as you step into movement? What soft tensions or sudden releases emerge? What lingers once the practice is complete? Noticing these subtleties builds interoceptive awareness, a sensitivity that allows patterns to emerge over time. Some find it useful to journal; others simply remember. Either way, a kind of internal compass forms, guiding choices in future sessions. Movement ceases to be linear exertion and becomes, instead, dialogue, improvisation, relationship.

One especially evocative practice is the threshold ritual. The idea is simple: establish a daily crossing point, a moment where you mark the shift from distraction into presence. Dawn, dusk, or some other turning point in the day. The ritual itself may be brief—a few breaths, a stretch coordinated with exhale, a mindful walk across familiar ground. What matters is not its duration but its regularity. Over time, such thresholds accumulate force, orienting the psyche, grounding the self, and reminding the practitioner that embodiment is not an afterthought but a mode of being.

Yet this vision must contend with the weight of cultural assumptions. Our society venerates measurable outcomes—miles logged, minutes timed, bodies shaped for the gaze. These have their uses, yes, but they obscure the subtler dimensions of wellbeing. This chapter pushes against that dominance, proposing another kind of success: not numbers on a chart but the capacity to listen and respond, to weave emotion and movement into coherence.

Examples bring this idea into sharper relief. Athletes sometimes describe training not as conquest but as conversation, a give-and-take between ambition and body's wisdom. Survivors of trauma often turn to somatic practices, discovering that healing arises not in recounting their stories alone but in gestures, breath, rhythm—movements that meet emotion where words cannot. Such accounts remind us that this is not theory alone but lived transformation.

In the end, this chapter offers both framework and practice for reclaiming movement as language, ritual, relationship. It does not promise perfection or performance but something more vital: the chance to inhabit the body with honesty, to discover how each step, each breath, each stretch might articulate an inner truth. Movement, seen in this way, ceases to be a burden or obligation. It becomes a ceremony of selfhood—messy, alive, evolving—through which resilience grows and wisdom takes root.

From Prescription to Ritual

Exercise, long prescribed as a functional task—an item on a checklist, a series of repetitions to fix or improve the body—has become an increasingly commodified, quantified, and at times alienating activity. Yet beneath this utilitarian framework lies a profound, often overlooked dimension: movement as a relational, expressive act that engages not only muscles but emotions, memories, and identity. To rewrite one's relationship to exercise is to shift from an externalised, performance-driven model toward an internal dialogue, a ritual that honours the body's intelligence and emotional complexity. This reframing is not a mere semantic tweak; it challenges the foundational assumptions that govern how society—and often individuals themselves—approach movement. The implications reach far beyond physical health, touching on mental wellbeing, self-awareness, and embodied agency.

Modern fitness culture frequently privileges measurable outcomes: weight lost, calories burned, personal records broken. While these metrics serve purposes within sport or rehabilitation, their dominance can distort the lived experience of movement, reducing it to a mechanical process detached from emotional nuance. This reductive perspective risks alienating those whose needs are not aligned with prevailing standards, fostering frustration, guilt, or disconnection. Moreover, such an approach often ignores the body's subtle signals—its rhythms, hesitations, and resonances—that hold vital clues about psychological states. Reclaiming movement as relational demands that we cultivate attentiveness to these signals, transforming exercise into a co-creative encounter with one's embodied self.

The transition from prescription to ritual begins with recognising movement as a form of communication—a language through which the body expresses feelings that may elude verbal articulation. This understanding finds resonance in somatic psychology and emerging neuroscientific research on interoception, which illuminate how bodily sensations underpin emotional experience and self-regulation. For example, a slow, mindful walk through nature can evoke a sense of calm and groundedness inaccessible through cognitive effort alone. Similarly, dance, with its expressive freedom, can surface repressed emotions, creating space for integration rather than avoidance. In these instances, movement is not a corrective measure but an exploratory ritual inviting presence, attunement, and acceptance.

This paradigm shift requires practical frameworks that empower individuals to tailor movement to their unique emotional landscape rather than conforming to generic prescriptions. *Mood-based movement maps*—a concept detailed in this chapter—offer a versatile tool, guiding choices that align physical modalities with current affective states. For instance, swimming's enveloping, fluid quality can support those navigating grief, while boxing's vigorous, grounded force may facilitate the healthy expression of anger. Such alignment honours the body's wisdom and resists the impulse to force movement to fit preordained templates. It also invites a richer, more compassionate engagement with oneself, mitigating the pressure to 'perform' or 'fix' and fostering exploration instead.

Central to this relational approach is cultivating *emotional feedback loops*—the practice of listening closely to somatic responses during and after movement. This involves noticing shifts in breath, muscle tone, heart rate, and affect, and reflecting on how these changes resonate with psychological states. By consistently attuning to these signals, practitioners build a nuanced, trustworthy dialogue with their bodies, which deepens self-knowledge and resilience. This iterative process transforms movement from a unilateral task into a responsive, adaptive practice—one that honours complexity rather than seeking oversimplified solutions.

The notion of a *daily movement threshold* ritual further concretises this approach by proposing an intentional, repeated crossing from mental preoccupation into embodied presence. Whether this takes the form of a brief breath-coordinated stretching sequence at dawn, a mindful walk that foregrounds sensation and environment, or a simple grounding gesture, such rituals act as anchors. They invite practitioners to inhabit their bodies fully at critical moments of the day, fostering continuity and integration amid the fragmentation characteristic of modern life. Over time, these threshold rituals cultivate a deepened capacity to move with intention and awareness, transcending the binary of doing versus being.

Rewriting exercise as relational ritual also entails critical reflection on broader sociocultural dynamics that shape our embodied practices. The prevailing fitness ethos often valorises discipline, control, and visible transformation, reinforcing ideals that may be alienating or exclusionary. Embracing movement as relational challenges these norms, advocating instead for inclusivity, emotional authenticity, and holistic wellbeing. This repositioning also highlights the ethical dimension of movement practice, inviting practitioners and coaches alike to foster environments where vulnerability and individual rhythms are respected, and where the goal is not uniformity but personal wholeness.

Throughout this chapter, real-world narratives enrich the conceptual discussion. Athletes who describe their craft as an ongoing conversation with their bodies, trauma survivors who access healing through somatic movement therapies, and dancers whose improvisations become embodied storytelling—all illustrate the transformative potential of reframing movement as relational ritual. These lived experiences attest to the profound shifts that occur when movement ceases to be a punitive or purely functional task and becomes a medium for emotional integration and self-expression.

Ultimately, *From Prescription to Ritual* is an invitation to reclaim movement as a deeply personal, emotionally intelligent practice—one that respects the body's wisdom, attends to its needs, and honours the complex interplay of mind, emotion, and flesh. By adopting this stance, readers are equipped not only to enhance physical vitality but also to nurture a more compassionate and embodied relationship with themselves. This shift holds promise not merely for individual transformation but for cultivating a culture that values movement as a sacred dialogue rather than a commercial or corrective transaction.

Mood-Based Movement Maps

The intimate relationship between emotion and movement has long been recognised across cultures and disciplines, yet modern exercise paradigms often neglect the nuanced ways in which specific physical practices resonate with particular emotional states. Mood-based movement maps represent an innovative framework that bridges this gap, guiding individuals to select movement styles attuned not merely to physical goals but to the emotional landscape they inhabit. This approach honours the body's implicit wisdom, acknowledging that different emotions call for distinct modes of embodiment—grief may seek the enveloping embrace of swimming, anger the directness of boxing, anxiety the gentle flow of tai chi. By cultivating this somatic-emotional alignment, movement becomes not only a means of physical engagement but a profound vehicle for emotional processing, regulation, and integration.

At the heart of mood-based movement maps is the recognition that emotions are embodied phenomena, manifesting through characteristic physiological patterns and movement tendencies. Contemporary affective neuroscience demonstrates that emotional states are closely intertwined with autonomic nervous system activity, muscle tone, and habitual postural patterns. For instance, sadness often correlates with a constricted chest and slowed movement, whereas anger is marked by increased muscle tension and expansive gestures. These embodied signatures provide valuable cues for selecting movement practices that either complement or recalibrate the prevailing mood. Ignoring these somatic-emotional correlations risks perpetuating dissonance between body and mind, whereas attuning movement to mood can enhance emotional resilience and self-awareness.

One instructive case is the use of swimming as a supportive practice for grief. The buoyancy and rhythmic immersion in water provide a cocooning environment that echoes the emotional need for containment and surrender. The repetitive, flowing strokes promote a meditative state, facilitating access to deeper layers of emotion while mitigating overwhelm. Qualitative studies of bereaved individuals engaging in aquatic therapy report reductions in anxiety and depressive symptoms, highlighting swimming's capacity to serve as a somatic refuge and emotional cleanser. The multisensory nature of water—the tactile, auditory, and proprioceptive inputs—engages the parasympathetic nervous system, fostering calm and emotional release.

Conversely, anger—a high-arousal emotion characterised by mobilised energy and readiness for action—finds an appropriate outlet in practices like boxing or martial arts. These modalities channel the intensity inherent in anger into structured, goal-directed movements, enabling catharsis without harm. Importantly, boxing's emphasis on rhythm, breath control, and precision also cultivates self-regulation within the expression of powerful affect. Neuroscientific investigations reveal that such practices engage motor planning areas and frontal networks implicated in impulse control, suggesting a dual process of release and regulation. Anecdotal reports from practitioners describe a heightened sense of agency and emotional clarity following sessions, underscoring the therapeutic potential of matching movement form to mood.

Anxiety, marked by heightened sympathetic arousal and disrupted interoceptive signalling, often responds favourably to slow, deliberate movement forms such as tai chi or qigong. These practices emphasise fluidity, breath synchronisation, and focused attention, effectively downregulating hypervigilance and restoring autonomic balance. Randomised controlled trials indicate that tai chi reduces anxiety symptoms and improves heart rate variability—a biomarker of parasympathetic tone—corroborating its mood-modulatory effects. Furthermore, the meditative quality of these movements fosters a mindful embodiment that helps individuals tolerate discomfort and uncertainty inherent in anxious states. Here, movement is a gentle dialogue with the body's alarm system, recalibrating its thresholds through paced engagement.

While these exemplars illustrate direct correspondences between emotion and movement style, mood-based movement maps also recognise the fluidity and complexity of human affect. Emotional states are rarely static; they fluctuate, overlap, and transform across time and context. Hence, a robust framework for mood-based movement incorporates principles of flexibility and responsiveness, encouraging individuals to cultivate a somatic literacy that discerns subtle shifts and selects accordingly. For example, a person navigating grief might alternate between swimming for containment and yoga for re-engagement with vitality, modulating practice in response to evolving emotional needs. Such dynamic attunement resists rigid prescriptions and invites personal experimentation, cultivating an embodied emotional intelligence.

Integrating mood-based movement maps into therapeutic and coaching settings requires sensitivity to cultural, developmental, and individual differences. Emotions and their somatic expressions are shaped by socialisation, trauma history, and personal narrative, complicating straightforward mappings. A client's embodied experience of anger, for instance, may differ widely from normative models, influenced by gender norms or repression. Skilled practitioners must therefore adopt a stance of curiosity and collaboration, co-creating movement prescriptions that respect the individual's unique somatic-emotional terrain. This relational approach enhances empowerment and avoids the pitfalls of mechanistic, one-size-fits-all programming.

Emerging technologies offer novel opportunities to refine and personalise mood-based movement maps. Wearable biosensors tracking heart rate variability, skin conductance, and motion patterns provide real-time data on physiological arousal and movement quality. When integrated with self-reported emotional states, such data can inform adaptive movement recommendations responsive to moment-to-moment affective shifts. Pilot studies in digital health demonstrate promising outcomes in mood regulation and adherence, though ethical considerations around data privacy and embodiment must be foregrounded. These innovations may eventually enable a more precise, embodied attunement between mood and movement, complementing traditional experiential knowledge.

Beyond individual benefit, mood-based movement maps hold potential for enhancing collective wellbeing. Group movement practices tailored to shared emotional states—such as grief circles incorporating gentle dance or anger release workshops utilising martial arts—can foster communal resilience and empathy. These embodied gatherings create somatic synchrony that amplifies emotional attunement, reinforcing social bonds and facilitating collective processing. Anthropological research on ritual movement supports this, illustrating how culturally embedded somatic practices serve as repositories of emotional regulation and social cohesion. Thus, mood-based movement extends its influence from personal integration to communal healing.

Critical voices caution against overly deterministic interpretations of emotion-movement correlations, warning that such models risk simplification and reification. Emotions are multifaceted phenomena with cognitive, cultural, and contextual dimensions that cannot be fully captured by somatic mappings alone. Moreover, some movement practices might trigger complex or contradictory emotional responses depending on individual history. This necessitates a tempered, reflexive application of mood-based movement maps, coupled with ongoing evaluation and openness to revision. The framework is best viewed as a flexible guide, a heuristic tool rather than a prescriptive formula.

In practice, adopting mood-based movement maps begins with cultivating *somatic attunement*—the capacity to notice bodily sensations associated with emotional states—and a vocabulary to describe these nuances. Journaling, mindful movement, and guided reflection support this development. From this foundation, individuals can experiment with movement modalities resonant with their mood profile, observing effects on emotional experience and wellbeing. Over time, this iterative process fosters a personalised movement ecology that honours the body's wisdom and nurtures emotional integration.

Mood-based movement maps represent a paradigm shift in how movement is conceptualised and utilised, moving beyond purely physical metrics toward a holistic, embodied engagement with emotion. By aligning movement style with emotional need, they empower individuals to harness the transformative potential of somatic practice—enhancing regulation, resilience, and self-understanding. This somatic-emotional synergy reframes movement from obligation or performance into an expressive, relational art form, vital for psychological health and enriched living.

Creating Emotional Feedback Loops

Listening to the body's whispers amidst movement often reveals more than muscle fatigue or cardiovascular exertion; it opens a gateway to the emotional self. Creating emotional feedback loops through movement practices is a transformative approach that teaches individuals to attune to somatic signals and trace the unfolding arc of emotions within their embodied experience. This process cultivates a dynamic conversation between mind and body, fostering inner trust, resilience, and psychological integration. Rather than treating movement as a mechanistic routine or solely a physical endeavour, it becomes an expressive dialogue—a potent medium through which emotional regulation and self-awareness are cultivated.

The foundation of emotional feedback loops lies in the principle that emotions are not abstract mental events but embodied phenomena, intrinsically linked to physiological states and movement patterns. Neuroscience and somatic psychology converge on the understanding that interoception—the perception of internal bodily sensations—constitutes a critical channel for emotional processing. When individuals learn to monitor subtle bodily cues such as breath depth, muscle tension, heart rate variability, or proprioceptive sensations during movement, they gain direct access to their emotional landscape. This somatic attunement, however, requires cultivation; it is neither automatic nor superficial but a skill developed through intentional practice and reflective observation.

Real-world applications of emotional feedback loops abound in disciplines such as somatic psychotherapy, dance therapy, and mindful movement practices like Feldenkrais or Alexander Technique. For example, in trauma-informed somatic therapy, clients are guided to notice how certain movements evoke sensations of safety, anxiety, or release, enabling them to map emotional terrain without relying solely on verbal articulation. This somatic 'mapmaking' supports clients in discerning which movement qualities soothe versus those that overwhelm, empowering them to calibrate their engagement and build resilience. Dance movement therapists often encourage clients to track the emotional shifts that arise from improvisational movement, using journaling or verbal reflection to create a feedback cycle between felt experience and conscious understanding.

Importantly, the emotional arc within a movement session is seldom linear; it ebbs and flows, mirrors complexity, and may evoke paradoxical responses. One might begin a practice feeling tense and restless, move into phases of cathartic release, and conclude with unexpected calm or insight. Observing and honouring these fluctuations without judgement or premature interpretation is essential. This open, non-linear engagement with emotional experience contrasts sharply with goal-oriented fitness paradigms, which prioritise performance outcomes over nuanced self-inquiry. The feedback loop approach reclaims movement as a container for emotional exploration, validation, and transformation.

A compelling case study emerges from research on mindful running, where practitioners report enhanced emotional clarity and stress reduction when encouraged to attend to breath rhythm, bodily sensations, and emotional tone during runs. Such practices foster a feedback loop wherein awareness of rising tension prompts subtle adjustments—slowing pace, deepening breath, or modulating posture—that in turn influence emotional states. This cyclical process builds embodied self-regulation, reducing reactivity and augmenting emotional resilience. The implications extend beyond running; they apply universally across movement modalities, highlighting the power of cultivating somatic dialogue.

Tracking emotional feedback during movement also entails cultivating language to describe nuanced bodily-affective states. The psychotherapeutic concept of *felt sense*, introduced by Eugene Gendlin, illuminates this process—whereby vague bodily sensations evolve into coherent emotional meanings through mindful attention. Practitioners encourage naming these experiences, whether 'tightness in the chest,' 'lightness in the limbs,' or 'a sinking feeling,' thereby bridging implicit bodily experience with explicit cognition. This translation strengthens the feedback loop, as articulating sensations fosters metacognitive reflection and deepens integration.

However, developing emotional feedback loops requires balancing attentive presence with safety. For individuals with histories of trauma or dysregulation, raw attention to bodily sensation without appropriate support can risk retraumatisation or overwhelm. Thus, scaffolding this practice within therapeutic or guided contexts—where pacing, containment, and grounding techniques are employed—is vital. Methods such as TRE (Tension and Trauma Release Exercises) or restorative yoga exemplify modalities that foster somatic awareness within gentle, regulated frameworks, facilitating safe engagement with challenging emotions.

Ethical considerations also surface in the application of emotional feedback loops, particularly regarding cultural variability in somatic-emotional expression. Movement and emotional norms differ across societies, and somatic signals carry culturally inflected meanings. Practitioners must therefore avoid universalising interpretations and instead adopt culturally humble approaches that respect individual and communal embodiments of emotion. Tailoring movement feedback to align with personal and cultural narratives enhances the relevance and accessibility of this practice.

Technological innovations increasingly contribute to refining emotional feedback loops. Wearable devices measuring physiological indices such as heart rate variability and galvanic skin response offer objective data points that complement subjective somatic awareness. Integrating these biosignals with self-reported emotional states enables more precise calibration of movement intensity and quality, fostering nuanced feedback cycles. For example, biofeedback-assisted yoga programs guide practitioners to modulate poses and breath to optimise autonomic balance. Nonetheless, reliance on technology must not supplant embodied listening; it should augment rather than replace human sensibility.

From a developmental perspective, emotional feedback loops echo the early formation of interoceptive and affective self-awareness in infancy, where caregivers attune to an infant's bodily signals to regulate distress and foster secure attachment. Re-engaging with this primary somatic dialogue in adulthood through movement offers a reparative avenue for disrupted regulation patterns. Movement thus becomes a vehicle for re-establishing foundational trust in one's body and emotions, counteracting disconnection or alienation that often characterises modern life.

Integrating emotional feedback loops into daily movement practice necessitates practical strategies. Starting sessions with a brief internal scan, noting current bodily-emotional states, sets a baseline for awareness. Throughout movement, practitioners can intermittently pause to check in with sensations and emotions, adjusting intensity or modality accordingly. After practice, reflective journaling or mindful contemplation consolidates insights, mapping shifts in mood or tension. Over time, this cyclical attentiveness fosters a deepening rapport with one's embodied emotional life, reinforcing self-trust.

This approach challenges prevalent cultural narratives that valorise disembodied productivity and rapid problem-solving, instead inviting a slower, more receptive mode of engagement with self. Movement becomes a sacred dialogue rather than a prescribed task—a space where vulnerability, curiosity, and self-compassion coalesce. Through cultivating emotional feedback loops, individuals transcend utilitarian notions of exercise and enter a realm where body and emotion co-create healing, insight, and resilience.

By anchoring movement in attentive somatic-emotional feedback, this practice aligns with contemporary integrative models of health that foreground mind-body reciprocity. It echoes foundational insights from pioneers such as Moshe Feldenkrais and Peter Levine, who emphasised somatic intelligence as central to wellbeing. Moreover, it resonates with emerging research underscoring the centrality of interoception in emotional regulation and mental health. Creating emotional feedback loops through movement thus stands as a vital, evidence-informed practice with profound implications for personal transformation and holistic health.

Ultimately, the cultivation of emotional feedback loops invites a radical reimagining of movement as a form of embodied dialogue. It demands patience, presence, and openness to the body's nuanced language, fostering an intimate partnership that builds inner trust and resilience. As practitioners learn to trace their emotional arcs through movement's dynamic contours, they reclaim a deeply personal, somatic wisdom—one that enriches not only their movement practice but the broader tapestry of emotional life.

The Daily Threshold

The start and end of a day are often punctuated by rituals—some deliberate, many habitual—that set the tone for how we engage with our environment and ourselves. Among these, a *daily movement threshold* ritual offers a powerful means of intentionally shifting from the fragmented, relentless mental chatter that saturates modern life into a grounded, embodied presence. This threshold is not merely about physical movement but represents a purposeful crossing into a state where body and mind coalesce, establishing a foundation of centred awareness from which the day can unfold or be concluded. Far from a simplistic fitness routine, this practice functions as a critical psychological and somatic boundary, marking a transition that cultivates clarity, emotional balance, and resilience.

The concept of a movement threshold ritual is rooted in the recognition that our bodies and minds are in constant dialogue, yet modern living often suppresses or bypasses this interaction. Our mornings might begin with a rush of thoughts, notifications, and anticipations, while evenings can be cluttered with residual stress and unresolved emotions. Movement, when framed as a deliberate rite of passage rather than a to-do list item, enables a recalibration—a somatic 'reset'—that reconnects us to ourselves beyond cognitive noise. This approach aligns with emerging research in embodied cognition, which emphasises that cognition is not confined to the brain but is distributed across the body's sensory and motor systems. The movement threshold ritual thus invites practitioners to harness this embodied cognition as a gateway into presence.

Consider the practice of Tai Chi or Qigong performed at dawn by practitioners worldwide. These slow, mindful sequences are not merely physical exercises but serve as *liminal rituals*—threshold crossings that gently dissolve the boundary between sleep and wakefulness, mindlessness and awareness. The flowing movements cultivate an internal focus that quiets mental clutter and invites sensory attunement to breath, posture, and subtle energy. The threshold is enacted through intention and repetition, creating a familiar embodied cue that signals the brain to shift modes. This transition is not trivial: it fosters neuroplasticity by reinforcing pathways associated with mindfulness and emotional regulation.

Similarly, the ritual of morning stretching or a brief session of restorative yoga exemplifies this threshold crossing in Western contexts. When practiced with intentionality—attending to the quality of movement, breath, and interoceptive sensations—these movements become more than physical routines. They serve as a bridge from abstract mental preoccupations into an integrated bodily experience. Anecdotal evidence from practitioners attests to how such rituals reduce anxiety, enhance focus, and foster a sense of agency. Moreover, framing movement as a threshold ritual counteracts the prevalent utilitarian mindset that values exercise primarily for external metrics such as calorie burn or aesthetics, instead positioning it as a gateway to psychological and emotional alignment.

Neuroscientific insights offer compelling explanations for the efficacy of threshold rituals. The brain's reticular activating system (RAS), responsible for regulating arousal and attention, responds powerfully to habitual sensory cues. A consistent movement threshold ritual can activate the RAS to facilitate alertness or calm, depending on the nature of the practice. This neurological tuning primes the individual's readiness to engage with the day or to release tension accumulated during wakefulness. In this light, the threshold ritual is not simply symbolic but foundational to optimizing cognitive and emotional functioning.

Yet, the power of the daily movement threshold lies equally in its accessibility and adaptability. It need not require elaborate or lengthy sessions; even a minute or two of conscious body movement can suffice if imbued with focused intention. For example, an individual might begin their day by standing barefoot, grounding through the feet, synchronising breath with gentle neck rolls or shoulder shrugs—movements that activate proprioception and parasympathetic regulation. This micro-ritual is a potent way to distinguish 'before' and 'after,' carving out psychological space that often remains elusive in fragmented modern schedules.

A critical element of the threshold practice is the cultivation of *ritualised attention*, an intentional focus on the movement's quality and felt experience. This differs markedly from mindless repetition or performance-driven exercise. Ritualised attention engages the parasympathetic nervous system, fostering a relaxation response that buffers stress and nurtures emotional regulation. It also cultivates *interoceptive awareness*, allowing individuals to sense and respond to subtle bodily states rather than reacting habitually or reflexively. Over time, this attentiveness fosters a deepened embodiment—a foundational component of mental health and well-being increasingly recognised in contemporary psychology.

Contrasting views might argue that embedding such ritual into daily life risks becoming another performance or obligation, especially in cultures saturated with productivity imperatives. However, when understood as an invitation rather than a mandate, the threshold ritual offers an opportunity to reclaim agency over one's embodied experience. It encourages individuals to design personal rituals that resonate with their unique rhythms and emotional landscapes rather than conforming to generic prescriptions. The empowerment found in this personalisation is transformative, fostering a sense of ownership over one's mental and emotional states.

Case studies from somatic psychotherapy illustrate the profound impact of integrating threshold rituals into daily routines. Clients who struggled with anxiety or dissociation often found that establishing a simple morning or evening movement practice anchored their sense of self and reduced symptom severity. One illustrative example involves a client who incorporated a brief standing meditation with slow arm movements each morning. This practice became a tangible 'landing place' in the swirling chaos of her thoughts, fostering resilience and emotional regulation. Therapists report that such rituals can act as early warning systems, enabling individuals to detect and modulate emotional shifts before they escalate.

The daily threshold ritual also bears ethical and cultural considerations. Movement practices and rituals carry cultural meanings that shape their emotional resonance and efficacy. Sensitivity to these dimensions is crucial when recommending or designing threshold rituals, ensuring respect for diverse embodied traditions and avoiding cultural appropriation. Embracing a culturally informed approach enhances the authenticity and sustainability of the practice.

Integrating technology, such as smartphone reminders or wearable biofeedback devices, may support the establishment and maintenance of threshold rituals. Yet, reliance on technology must be balanced with cultivating intrinsic motivation and embodied presence. The goal is to transcend external prompts and develop an internal somatic compass that naturally signals the daily threshold.

Ultimately, the daily movement threshold ritual reclaims a neglected space between mind and body, action and presence. It transforms movement from a mere physical act into a meaningful, embodied passage—a deliberate crossing that initiates psychological readiness and emotional attunement. By embedding this practice into the fabric of daily life, individuals cultivate a foundation of centredness that not only enhances well-being but also enriches every subsequent engagement with the world. This ritualised threshold offers a timeless antidote to the fragmented, distracted condition of contemporary existence, reminding us that presence is both a practice and a passage—one that begins with the simple, profound act of moving with intention.

Chapter 10
A New Psychology Begins in Motion

The future of psychology, if it is to remain relevant to the fullness of human experience, requires nothing short of recalibration. Not a minor adjustment of technique, but a sweeping shift—one that moves beyond the static confines of the consulting room and welcomes the body, with all its sensations, gestures, and rhythms, into the very centre of therapeutic practice. This chapter, *A New Psychology Begins in Motion*, lays the groundwork for such a transformation: a psychology where movement is not decorative, not supplemental, but a primary mode of healing, integration, and growth. Contemporary approaches—somatic experiencing, sensorimotor psychotherapy, embodied coaching—already point the way, showing us that the psyche cannot be disentangled from the living, breathing, moving organism in which it resides. To understand the mind fully, we must listen to its kinetic speech, its somatic dialects, the visceral murmurings beneath thought.

This embodied turn is no mere elaboration of methods; it is a challenge to the cultural hierarchies that govern how we conceive health. Ours is a society enthralled by numbers, obsessed with standardised outcomes, with metrics that reduce vitality to neat graphs and scores. Schools, workplaces, even clinics often mirror this fragmented outlook, stripping wellbeing of its organic messiness. To rewire such a culture demands more than policy reform—it requires reimagining the very environments where we learn, labour, and heal. Imagine spaces where the body's wisdom is not tolerated on the margins but honoured at the centre, where movement is embedded into daily life as necessity rather than extracurricular luxury, where the long-standing split between mind and body gives way to a more seamless whole.

At the heart of this vision lies a strikingly simple yet radical imperative: to inhabit our aliveness. Not to chase abstract ideals of "mental health" detached from lived sensation, but to meet ourselves as responsive, emotional, continually moving beings. Such a shift asks for presence, real presence—the kind that notices emotion in a bent spine or restless hand, that acknowledges how rhythm and gesture shape our inner life, and that dares to lean into discomfort rather than bypass it. Aliveness is not a trophy to be won, but an ongoing unfolding: sensation, feeling, movement interweaving into the raw texture of selfhood.

To sustain such a shift, we must cultivate what might be called movement literacy. This is not the jargon of fitness regimes, but a deeper fluency in how the body expresses and receives meaning. Such literacy serves not only personal growth—emotional, spiritual—but also the social fabric. It sharpens empathy, refines attunement, and enables a level of communication that sidesteps words altogether. It reminds us that rituals of collective movement, whether in dance, pilgrimage, or everyday gestures of care, can bind communities more effectively than rhetoric ever could. In this sense, movement is more than exercise; it is language—subtle, multi-layered, profoundly human.

What follows in this chapter is an invitation to readers: to see how therapeutic practice is reshaped when movement is integrated at its core. The arguments draw from clinical evidence, emerging science, and imaginative vision. Taken together, they suggest a future where psychology is not simply spoken or analysed but lived—embodied, enacted, in motion. This is no cosmetic change of method. It is a reorientation, almost a revolution: a summons to awaken the body's wisdom, to restore its rightful place at the centre of mental life, and to embrace a psychology that, quite literally, moves with us.

Toward an Embodied Therapeutics

The traditional confines of psychotherapy, grounded predominantly in talk and cognition, are no longer sufficient to address the complex, embodied nature of human distress and healing. *Toward an Embodied Therapeutics* signals a profound recalibration in the mental health field—one that insists movement and somatic experience must be integrated at the core of therapeutic practice. This shift reflects a growing recognition that psychological wounds and emotional dysregulation manifest not only in thought patterns or language but through the lived body: posture, gesture, breath, and implicit motor patterns. To move beyond symptomatic treatment and foster genuine transformation, psychotherapy must embrace the body as a vital participant in healing.

Among the pioneering modalities advancing this embodied approach are somatic experiencing, sensorimotor psychotherapy, and embodied coaching, each offering distinct yet complementary frameworks. Somatic experiencing, developed by Peter Levine, centres on resolving trauma by attending to bodily sensations and restoring the nervous system's capacity to self-regulate. It foregrounds the body's innate wisdom, inviting clients to notice micro-movements and subtle shifts that signal safety or threat. This methodology reframes trauma not solely as a cognitive or emotional event but as an incomplete biological response requiring somatic completion through movement and sensation.

Sensorimotor psychotherapy, founded by Pat Ogden, builds on similar principles but integrates attachment theory and cognitive interventions alongside somatic awareness. It explicitly connects movement patterns with relational schemas, highlighting how habitual bodily postures encapsulate adaptive or maladaptive survival strategies shaped by early experiences. Sensorimotor therapy actively utilises movement to recalibrate these patterns, creating pathways for new embodied narratives that support emotional resilience and relational attunement. This approach underscores how the body is not a passive vessel but an active agent in psychological processes, capable of both encoding trauma and fostering healing.

Embodied coaching further extends this paradigm into the realms of performance, leadership, and everyday wellness. It emphasises *presence*—the capacity to inhabit one's body fully and respond fluidly to shifting internal and external conditions. Through movement-based inquiry, embodied coaching cultivates heightened somatic literacy, enabling individuals to detect subtle signals, manage stress, and harness emotional energy constructively. Unlike traditional coaching models that often privilege cognitive strategies and goal-setting, embodied coaching insists on *dialogue* with the body as a source of insight and transformation.

These embodied therapeutic modalities challenge the dominance of mind-centred psychology by validating the body's role as a site of knowledge and agency. They respond to a growing body of neurobiological research demonstrating how trauma and emotion are deeply intertwined with sensorimotor systems. The vagus nerve, for instance, acts as a critical conduit linking emotional regulation with physiological states, while mirror neurons and interoceptive pathways reveal how body-based empathy shapes social cognition. Ignoring these embodied dimensions risks superficial interventions that may alleviate symptoms without addressing root causes.

Yet, the integration of movement into therapy is not without conceptual tensions. Some practitioners raise concerns about the risk of overemphasising somatic techniques at the expense of verbal processing or cognitive insight. Others question how to maintain rigorous therapeutic boundaries when physical movement becomes a modality for emotional expression. Such debates highlight the necessity for embodied therapeutics to remain integrative, drawing on multiple modalities rather than privileging one over another. Movement must complement, not replace, the full spectrum of psychological inquiry.

Real-world applications of embodied therapeutics illustrate its transformative potential. For example, trauma survivors who have struggled with dissociation often report breakthroughs when therapy incorporates guided movement or breathwork, enabling reconnection with bodily sensations that had been inaccessible. In clinical settings, sensorimotor techniques have been shown to reduce PTSD symptoms and improve emotional regulation more effectively than talk therapy alone in some cases. In leadership development, embodied coaching fosters enhanced presence and interpersonal attunement, leading to improved decision-making and relational dynamics.

The ethical dimensions of embodied therapeutics also demand attention. Working with the body requires sensitivity to power dynamics, consent, and cultural contexts. Therapists must be attuned to how movement interventions might trigger vulnerability or retraumatization and must cultivate skills in holding and containing somatic experience. This necessitates specialised training and ongoing supervision to ensure safe and effective practice.

Looking ahead, the integration of movement into psychotherapy signals a paradigm shift that aligns with broader trends in health and wellness towards holistic, person-centred care. It invites a reconsideration of what it means to be human—complex, embodied, and dynamically interconnected with one's environment. This new psychology honours the body not merely as an object to be fixed but as a living archive of experience, a compass for emotional navigation, and a wellspring of resilience.

Embodied therapeutics thus offers a roadmap for healing that is as much about *being* as it is about *doing*. It encourages therapists and clients alike to listen deeply—to the body's rhythms, tensions, and releases—and to cultivate a relational dance that transcends words. In embracing movement as a vital therapeutic language, psychology opens new possibilities for integration, empowerment, and wholeness.

Rewiring the Culture of Health

The prevailing culture of health within modern institutions is dominated by a relentless emphasis on quantification—steps counted, calories burned, heart rates monitored, and biometric scores aggregated. While these metrics offer valuable insights, their primacy often obscures a more profound truth: *health is a lived, embodied experience that cannot be reduced to numbers alone.* The imperative to rewire this culture, especially within schools, clinics, and workplaces, is no longer a matter of preference but necessity. As sedentary lifestyles and stress-related disorders surge, the limitations of a metrics-driven paradigm become increasingly evident, prompting a call for environments designed around *meaningful movement*—spaces that prioritise the quality of bodily engagement over mere numerical targets.

The institutional fixation on metrics emerged from a laudable impulse to standardise and democratise health interventions. Public health campaigns and corporate wellness programmes have sought to mobilise populations through easily measurable goals, such as the ubiquitous ten-thousand steps daily benchmark. However, this reductionist framework often fails to capture the *emotional, social, and psychological dimensions of movement.* It can inadvertently alienate individuals whose lived realities do not conform to idealised norms, thereby reinforcing inequities and neglecting the diverse ways people experience their bodies. Moreover, the dominance of metrics risks commodifying movement as a performance to be optimized rather than a relational, restorative process integral to human thriving.

Schools represent a critical arena for reimagining movement culture. Traditional physical education models frequently prioritise competitive sports and standardised fitness assessments, sidelining the potential for movement to foster *embodiment, creativity, and emotional regulation.* Progressive educational frameworks have begun to introduce movement practices that attend to *mindfulness, play, and somatic awareness*, recognising these as foundational to cognitive and social development. For instance, programs incorporating yoga, dance, and free-form movement enable students to cultivate a nuanced connection with their bodies, which correlates with improved attention, stress resilience, and interpersonal skills. Such interventions challenge the narrow view of exercise as a mechanical task and instead position it as a *holistic modality* supporting well-rounded growth.

In clinical settings, the entrenched focus on diagnostics and outcome metrics similarly constrains the integration of movement as a therapeutic ally. Yet, disciplines such as physiotherapy, occupational therapy, and increasingly, psychotherapy are embracing *embodied approaches* that acknowledge how movement patterns reflect and shape psychological states. Clinics that incorporate movement into treatment protocols attend not just to symptom reduction but to restoring agency, rhythm, and flow. For example, trauma-informed care frameworks now often include somatic experiencing or dance/movement therapy, recognising that healing unfolds through the body's capacity to release, regulate, and re-engage with sensation. This transition towards embodied therapeutics calls for institutional redesigns that support *safe, accessible, and varied movement opportunities* as integral components of health infrastructure.

Workplaces, long synonymous with prolonged sitting and mental fatigue, offer fertile ground for cultivating a culture of movement attuned to human flourishing. While wellness initiatives tend to centre on discrete interventions—standing desks, scheduled exercise breaks, or fitness challenges—the transformative potential lies in *embedding movement into the very architecture and social fabric of work life.* Biophilic design principles, for instance, encourage the integration of natural elements and movement pathways that invite spontaneous physical engagement. Additionally, organisational cultures that normalise micro-movements, collective stretch breaks, or walking meetings disrupt the static postures associated with chronic stress and musculoskeletal disorders. By recalibrating workplace norms to value *movement as a means of cognitive refreshment and relational connection*, organisations can enhance employee wellbeing and productivity synergistically.

Rewiring the culture of health thus demands a *paradigm shift from mechanistic, metric-driven models to relational, meaning-infused practices.* This does not entail abandoning measurement but reframing it within a broader context that honours subjective experience and diversity. Metrics must serve as *tools to inform compassionate, personalised movement practices rather than as rigid benchmarks.* Achieving this requires multi-level collaboration—policy makers fostering environments conducive to movement equity, educators adopting curricula that celebrate somatic intelligence, healthcare providers integrating embodied modalities, and employers designing work systems that honour the body's rhythms.

Real-world exemplars illuminate the feasibility and impact of this shift. The Finnish education system's incorporation of regular movement breaks and outdoor play correlates with improved student engagement and health outcomes. Integrative clinics in Scandinavia and parts of the US are pioneering movement-based psychotherapies with demonstrable benefits in trauma recovery. Companies such as Patagonia have restructured workspaces and schedules to prioritise employee movement and social connection, witnessing reductions in burnout and absenteeism. These models underscore that *movement-centred cultures are not utopian fantasies but attainable frameworks* grounded in evidence and humanistic values.

Nonetheless, the transition encounters resistance from entrenched interests invested in current paradigms and the inertia of institutional routines. The commodification of health through wearable technologies and commercial fitness industries often reinforces a transactional view of movement, obscuring its relational and ecological dimensions. Moreover, disparities in access to safe, welcoming movement spaces pose ethical challenges that demand systemic interventions to prevent further marginalisation.

Addressing these complexities calls for ongoing critical reflection and adaptive strategies. It involves recognising movement as a *dynamic dialogue between body, mind, and environment*—a source of agency, identity, and community. Cultivating environments that honour this dialogue requires rethinking architectural design, social policies, educational priorities, and clinical practices through a lens that centres *movement's qualitative richness alongside quantitative assessment.*

Ultimately, rewiring the culture of health is an invitation to reclaim movement as a vital expression of *aliveness and belonging.* It demands that institutions become facilitators of embodied experience rather than mere arbiters of numeric standards. This transformation promises not only improved physical health but also the revitalisation of emotional, social, and spiritual dimensions of human life, forging a more integrated and compassionate future.

Living Inside Your Aliveness

The prevailing discourse on mental wellness often anchors itself in abstract ideals—an imagined state of perpetual calm, balance, and control that many find elusive, if not alienating. This conceptualisation risks reducing the human experience to a checklist of symptoms to be managed rather than embracing the complex reality of living as a *responsive, emotional, and moving organism.* To live *inside your aliveness* is to reject static definitions of health and instead inhabit a fluid, embodied existence that honours the full spectrum of affective experience and somatic presence. Such a perspective demands a fundamental reorientation of how we understand ourselves, mental health, and the body-mind relationship.

Contemporary mental health paradigms have largely been shaped by biomedical models that prioritise symptom alleviation and cognitive regulation. While these approaches have their place, they tend to fragment experience—separating mind from body, emotion from action. By contrast, emerging somatic psychologies, embodied therapies, and integrative neuroscience propose that *mental wellness is inseparable from bodily vitality and movement.* The body is not merely a vessel for the mind but a primary site of knowing and feeling. Emotions manifest in muscular tension, posture, breath patterns, and kinetic rhythms, providing rich somatic data about our internal state. To live inside one's aliveness is to cultivate *somatic awareness* that informs a responsive engagement with life, rather than striving for an unattainable ideal of emotional stasis.

This embodied perspective challenges the cultural narrative that frames mental wellness as a goal of mental control or absence of distress. It acknowledges that emotions—ranging from joy and love to grief and rage—are vital signals guiding adaptive action. For example, anger, often pathologised, can be understood as a catalyst for boundary-setting and empowerment when embodied and expressed authentically. Similarly, grief invites slow, somatic processing that cannot be hurried or intellectualised away. To deny these emotional currents is to estrange oneself from the natural fluctuations of aliveness. The work, therefore, is not to suppress or manage emotions in a detached manner but to *engage them through the body's inherent wisdom.*

Real-world applications of this embodied ethos appear in therapeutic modalities such as somatic experiencing, which traces trauma as a dysregulation of the nervous system and uses body-based interventions to restore resilience. Sensorimotor psychotherapy integrates talk therapy with mindful attention to bodily sensations and movement patterns, helping clients reconnect fragmented aspects of self. Embodied coaching frameworks extend these principles beyond pathology, encouraging clients to develop movement fluency as a resource for creativity, presence, and relational attunement. These approaches demonstrate that *mental wellness arises from the dynamic interplay between sensation, movement, and emotion*, rather than abstract cognitive constructs alone.

Moreover, living inside your aliveness invites reconsideration of everyday habits that shape mental states. Modern lifestyles often impose sedentary routines, technological immersion, and mental multitasking that diminish bodily engagement and fragment attention. This disconnect can exacerbate anxiety, depression, and a pervasive sense of alienation. Conversely, practices that foreground embodied presence—such as mindful walking, conscious breathing, dance, or yoga—activate the parasympathetic nervous system, modulate stress responses, and foster integration between body and mind. The intentional cultivation of *embodied rituals* offers a potent antidote to the disembodied mental wellness ideals prevalent in contemporary culture.

Crucially, this perspective foregrounds *responsivity* rather than rigidity. To live inside one's aliveness is to develop an attunement to internal signals that guide adaptive responses to shifting circumstances. This requires cultivating curiosity toward bodily sensations and emotional states, cultivating an internal dialogue that listens rather than judges. The process is deeply individual and resists universal prescriptions. For some, vigorous movement may ignite vitality; for others, restorative stillness holds the key. The capacity to discern what the body-mind system needs in any moment exemplifies a profound form of self-trust and resilience.

This reorientation also carries ethical and social implications. Embracing embodied aliveness entails recognising the embeddedness of individuals within relational and environmental contexts. Our mental and emotional states are shaped by social dynamics, cultural narratives, and ecological conditions. Practices that foster embodied presence can thus serve as portals to deeper social connection, empathy, and ecological attunement. Movements such as community dance, somatic group therapy, and nature immersion exemplify how living inside our aliveness can extend outward to cultivate collective wellbeing.

Nevertheless, integrating this embodied paradigm into mainstream mental health and daily life encounters resistance. Dominant institutions and commercial wellness industries often prefer simplified, commodifiable solutions that fit neatly into consumer lifestyles or clinical protocols. The nuanced, iterative, and sometimes messy work of embodied integration challenges quick fixes and demands sustained, attentive practice. Yet, as research increasingly underscores the centrality of embodiment to psychological health, the imperative to shift paradigms grows more urgent.

Ultimately, *living inside your aliveness* is an invitation to reclaim the fullness of human experience beyond reductionist definitions of mental wellness. It demands an embrace of complexity, a willingness to feel deeply and move authentically, and a commitment to cultivating presence through the body's wisdom. This embodied aliveness offers a foundation for mental, emotional, and relational flourishing that is not only more attainable but more deeply human. To inhabit this paradigm is to rediscover what it means to be truly alive.

A New Movement Literacy

Movement literacy remains an overlooked dimension of human intelligence, overshadowed by the dominant prioritisation of cognitive and verbal skills in education, healthcare, and society at large. Yet, movement fluency—our capacity to move with awareness, adaptability, and expressive nuance—is foundational not only to physical health but also to emotional regulation, spiritual connection, and social communication. The imperative to cultivate a *new movement literacy* stems from an evolving understanding that human flourishing is intrinsically embodied, and that mastery of movement language enriches all facets of our lives. This article argues for a profound revaluation of movement as a core form of intelligence, essential for navigating the complexities of the modern world.

Traditional notions of fitness often reduce movement to quantifiable metrics: strength, endurance, flexibility, speed. While such markers hold undeniable value, they reflect only a fraction of what it means to move intelligently. Movement fluency encompasses *kinesthetic awareness*, the ability to sense and interpret bodily sensations; *motor adaptability*, the capacity to respond to dynamic environments; and *expressive communication*, the subtle language of gesture, posture, and rhythm through which we relate to others. These capacities underpin emotional attunement, empathy, and even spiritual presence. For example, dance therapy illustrates how nuanced movement patterns facilitate emotional processing and interpersonal connection, while martial arts cultivate discipline alongside mindful responsiveness. This breadth of movement literacy exceeds the domain of physical fitness to engage the *whole person.*

Neuroscientific research lends empirical weight to the centrality of movement in cognitive and emotional functioning. Mirror neuron systems, implicated in empathy and social cognition, activate through observation and imitation of movement, underpinning our ability to resonate with others' emotional states. Sensorimotor integration facilitates the brain's coordination of perception, action, and emotion, supporting fluid engagement with complex social contexts. Conversely, movement restriction or disembodiment correlates with emotional dysregulation and social withdrawal, as seen in conditions such as depression and trauma. These findings compel a shift from viewing movement as ancillary to mental processes toward recognising it as an *integral medium* of emotional and social intelligence.

Education systems exemplify the need for a movement literacy renaissance. Increasingly sedentary classrooms, emphasising standardised testing and screen time, compromise children's embodied development, limiting opportunities to explore spatial awareness, balance, and interoceptive signals. Emerging pedagogical models—such as *embodied learning*, *kinesthetic classrooms*, and *movement integration*—demonstrate enhanced attention, creativity, and emotional resilience among students. Programs that incorporate yoga, improvisational theatre, or outdoor play illustrate how movement cultivates neural plasticity, stress regulation, and social cohesion. To foster a new movement literacy, curricula must expand beyond physical education as isolated 'gym time' to embrace movement as a *daily modality of learning* that nurtures emotional and relational capacities.

In clinical settings, movement literacy informs integrative approaches that honour the body's wisdom alongside psychological insight. Somatic psychotherapies harness movement to access implicit memories and reshape entrenched patterns, while embodied coaching encourages clients to develop *movement vocabularies* attuned to personal values and goals. Movement analysis tools, such as Laban Movement Analysis, offer frameworks to decode the emotional subtext of posture and gesture, enriching therapeutic attunement. These embodied methods challenge Cartesian dualism and medicalised reductionism by foregrounding movement as a *language of healing* and self-discovery. They exemplify how cultivating movement fluency can deepen emotional insight and foster holistic wellbeing.

Movement literacy also plays a vital role in spiritual practice, where the body serves as a vessel for transcendent experience and ritual embodiment. Practices like qigong, Sufi whirling, and indigenous dance demonstrate how cultivated movement fosters states of flow, presence, and connection to collective meaning. These traditions underscore that movement fluency is not merely functional but *transformative*, enabling practitioners to navigate altered states of consciousness and foster inner integration. Incorporating such embodied practices into contemporary wellness expands the notion of intelligence to include *spiritual embodiment*, a dimension often neglected in secular health discourses.

Social intelligence is similarly grounded in movement fluency. Nonverbal communication—facial expression, eye contact, posture, proxemics—constitutes a rich, largely unconscious exchange that shapes interpersonal rapport and group dynamics. Effective social interaction depends on subtle movement attunement, synchronisation, and rhythmic coordination. For example, research on *interactional synchrony* demonstrates how shared movement patterns promote trust and cooperation. Dance, theatre, and sports exemplify communal movement literacy, creating social bonds and cultural identity through embodied practice. Thus, cultivating movement fluency enhances not only individual agency but collective cohesion.

The call for a new movement literacy is timely given the contemporary challenges of pervasive sedentism, digital distraction, and emotional fragmentation. Reclaiming movement as an intelligent, expressive, and integrative practice offers a pathway to counterbalance the mechanisation of human experience. It invites us to develop *a richer vocabulary of bodily presence* that supports emotional agility, spiritual depth, and social harmony. Practical cultivation of this literacy involves mindful movement practices, cross-disciplinary education, and inclusive access to embodied arts and therapies.

To this end, institutions and communities must reimagine spaces and policies that nurture movement fluency across the lifespan.

Workplaces can incorporate movement breaks that focus on somatic awareness rather than calorie burning; schools can embed creative movement as foundational to curriculum; healthcare systems can integrate embodied assessments and interventions; urban planning can prioritise walkability and communal movement zones. These shifts require systemic commitment but promise profound returns in public health, social wellbeing, and cultural vitality.

In essence, developing a new movement literacy entails more than learning exercises or mastering techniques. It is a transformative engagement with the self as a moving, feeling organism embedded in relational and ecological contexts. This fluency cultivates *embodied wisdom*—an intuitive, adaptive intelligence that transcends words and metrics. It reconnects us with our inherent capacity to move meaningfully through the world, shaping not only our bodies but our emotions, spirits, and communities. To cultivate this literacy is to reclaim a fundamental dimension of human life, essential for thriving in complexity and change.

Conclusion
The Intelligence Beneath Your Feet

To imagine emotional intelligence as purely a matter of the mind is to miss the deeper register in which it actually unfolds—the wisdom carried in the body's movements, the wordless lexicon of gesture, rhythm, and breath that shapes our sense of self and our connection to others. This closing chapter suggests a fundamental reorientation: emotional literacy is not confined to verbal finesse or reflective thought but lived physically, expressed in the cadence of a walk, the reach of a stretch, the sway of a torso, the sudden eruption of a sprint. The journey charted in these pages has not been towards a catalogue of techniques so much as a way of inhabiting the world: an embodied practice in which emotion takes form at the intersection of body, mind, and environment. Perhaps, then, the next breakthrough in one's emotional life will not be unearthed by further rumination, but through the kinaesthetic intelligence hidden in ordinary movements.

This notion of embodied emotionality is neither abstract nor esoteric. It is immediate, accessible, and deeply practical. Consider the dancer whose flowing improvisation unknots inner tension, or the runner whose steady rhythm clears the fog of indecision, or even the office worker who rises for a stretch that disrupts the slow build of stress. These are not curiosities but expressions of an intimate tie between movement and emotional processing. Neuroscientific findings affirm this: sensorimotor networks braid bodily sensation with affect, and the autonomic nervous system—so often overlooked—shapes both mood and posture in tandem. The point is inescapable. Movement is not an adjunct to mental health, but a primary route to awareness, regulation, and change.

Over the course of this book, movement has been considered as a means of integration, as a form of communication, and even as ritual or quiet defiance. Now, the call is to take this understanding inward, to wear it as a continuous practice rather than an intellectual concept. What is required is not a checklist of exercises but a cultivated openness to the body's subtle messages. This shift from technique to stance parallels the insights of somatic therapies, which privilege embodied experience above cognitive control, reminding us that genuine insight often arrives as sensation before it ever becomes articulated thought.

The implications ripple outward, beyond personal growth. Our cultural inheritance has long privileged the intellect, sidelining the wisdom of the body. Mainstream models of mental health too frequently marginalise somatic knowing, defaulting to talk or pharmacology while neglecting movement and sensation. This chapter therefore issues a broader provocation: to reshape how we conceive of wellbeing. Imagine schools where movement-rich practices foster resilience, workplaces designed to interrupt stress through micro-movements rather than extended stillness, and clinics where somatic attunement is not exotic but expected.

Such collective change amplifies the private work of reclaiming emotional agency through embodied practice. What emerges is the dissolution of rigid boundaries between thought, feeling, and action, replaced by a more fluid reciprocity. Emotional insight ceases to appear as sudden revelation; it becomes the by-product of ongoing engagement, the natural evolution of a body in motion. This reframing asks for patience, a willingness to proceed gently, recognising that fluency in this realm develops over years, sculpted by history and circumstance as much as by discipline.

Practical entry points exist: cultivating small rituals of mindful movement, attending closely to the body's feedback, experimenting with varied forms—dance, yoga, martial arts, breathwork—according to personal resonance. Movement here does not need to be strenuous or spectacular; sometimes a simple shift in posture, a hand unclenching, or even an attentive stillness can unlock new emotional possibilities. The aim is to form a relationship with the body as confidant and guide, not as an object to be monitored or subdued.

In the end, the invitation is to inhabit a revised understanding of emotional intelligence—one that regards the body not as accessory but as primary site of knowing. The radicality lies less in complexity than in its disarming simplicity: the body already speaks. Each step, bend, or gesture is a conversation with that intelligence, an opening through which understanding can flow without words. To attend to this dimension is to embrace a richer, more integrated existence, where emotional literacy is not merely thought about but felt, moved, and lived in the quiet intelligence beneath our feet.

Summarizes the journey not as a set of techniques, but a way of being:

The conventional wisdom surrounding emotional intelligence situates it firmly in the realm of cognition, relegating the body to a passive vessel for mental processes. Yet, this perspective overlooks a fundamental truth: emotional literacy is not merely a faculty of the mind but an embodied capacity, continuously enacted through movement and physical expression. This subchapter pivots the reader's understanding from treating emotional awareness as a discrete set of intellectual skills to embracing it as a *way of being*—one lived through the subtle dynamics of posture, gesture, breath, and motion. The challenge posed here is not to learn more techniques or add routines but to inhabit an integrated state where body and emotion coalesce into a fluent, responsive dialogue.

The synthesis of emotion and movement runs deeper than popular notions of "mind-body connection." Neuroscientific research illuminates how sensorimotor circuits and affective networks are inseparable, each shaping the other in real time. Emotions manifest somatically before being translated into language or thought; the quiver of anxiety, the surge of joy, the slump of grief—these are first and foremost physical phenomena. When we view emotional literacy through this embodied lens, we acknowledge that *feeling* is enacted in the very architecture of our movement patterns. Our habitual ways of moving become emotional signatures, and our ability to modulate these patterns translates into emotional agility.

Real-world applications abound. In clinical settings, somatic therapies that foreground bodily awareness have demonstrated profound efficacy in resolving trauma and regulating affect. Meanwhile, practitioners across disciplines—from dance to martial arts to breathwork—describe how movement cultivates an intuitive emotional intelligence that defies verbal explanation. These lived experiences underscore a critical insight: emotional breakthroughs often emerge not from deliberate rumination but from shifts in bodily state—an uncoiling stretch, a grounding step, an expressive sway. Movement becomes not just an adjunct to emotion but a primary mode through which emotional self-understanding is accessed and transformed.

This embodied approach also disrupts reductive binaries that pit mind against body or reason against feeling. Instead, it proposes a holistic model where *presence*—the capacity to be fully attentive to one's felt experience—is cultivated through physical engagement. Such presence deepens our capacity for emotional nuance, allowing us to notice shifts in mood before they crystallise into distress or reactivity. This continuous feedback loop between body and affect cultivates resilience, making it possible to navigate complex emotional landscapes with greater ease and sophistication.

A practical implication is the invitation to reframe everyday movement not as mechanistic or functional but as an opportunity for emotional attunement. Simple acts—standing, walking, stretching—can be consciously oriented towards an internal dialogue, becoming ritualised moments of self-connection. This shift from doing *to* movement towards being *in* movement cultivates a transformative relationship with the body as a trusted emotional guide rather than an object of control or scrutiny.

Importantly, this subchapter confronts the cultural tendency to intellectualise or commodify emotional work, which risks alienating the embodied self. It challenges readers to relinquish the pursuit of neat conceptual frameworks in favour of *experiential fluency*, a lived competence in listening to and expressing emotional states through movement. This is a call to rediscover the body's ancient, innate wisdom—a form of knowing that is tactile, dynamic, and immediate.

The final provocation is both simple and profound: *what if your next emotional breakthrough isn't located in the labyrinth of your mind but in the fluid arc of your next step, the unfurling of a stretch, the rhythmic sway of your breath, or the energetic release of a sprint?* To entertain this possibility is to open oneself to a richer, more embodied way of engaging with emotions—one that honours the whole person rather than fragmenting experience into abstract categories.

This embodied literacy reframes emotional health as an ongoing practice rather than a fixed destination, a continual attunement to the intelligence beneath our feet and the movement coursing through our being. As such, it invites a profound recalibration of self-understanding, offering a path toward emotional integration that is felt, lived, and expressed in every movement we make. The journey is not a prescription to follow but a *state to inhabit*—a dynamic conversation between body and emotion that holds the potential for deeper insight, healing, and aliveness.

About the Author

Dr. Adrian Vale is a somatic psychologist, movement theorist, and lecturer with a deep-rooted passion for exploring the living dialogue between body and mind. Holding a doctorate in embodied cognition and with over a decade of experience in integrative therapy and movement facilitation, Dr. Vale has guided individuals and communities through transformative practices that meld neuroscience, anthropology, and ritual into everyday motion. Drawing inspiration from both ancient wisdom and cutting-edge research, Adrian writes with warmth, intellectual rigor, and profound insight—exactly the blend readers will find at the heart of Move for Mood. As a mindful-living advocate akin to authors like Evelyn Blythe and Elena Khurana featured on Mindful Pages Publishers, Dr. Vale's work bridges academic depth and soulful resonance, positioning them as the ideal voice for this genre.

www.ingramcontent.com/pod-product-compliance
Lightning Source LLC
Chambersburg PA
CBHW031350230926
51848CB00002B/465